happy gut,
happy mind

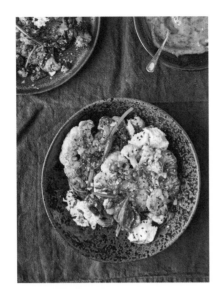

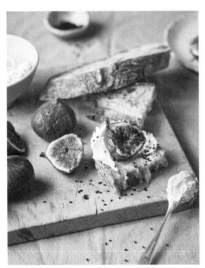

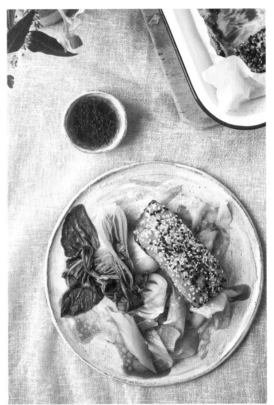

happy gut, happy mind

How to feel good from within

eve kalinik

PIATKUS

PIATKUS

First published in Great Britain in 2020 by Piatkus
1 3 5 7 9 10 8 6 4 2

A CIP catalogue record for this book
is available from the British Library.

ISBN 978-0-349-42377-7

Printed and bound in Great Britain by Bell and Bain Ltd, Glasgow

All photography © Nassima Rothacker
Food stylist: Rosie Ramsden
Book design: D. R. ink
Editors: Maggie Ramsden and Jillian Stewart

Papers used by Piatkus are from well-managed forests and other responsible sources.

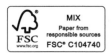

Piatkus
An imprint of
Little, Brown Book Group
Carmelite House
50 Victoria Embankment
London EC4Y 0DZ

An Hachette UK Company
www.hachette.co.uk

www.littlebrown.co.uk

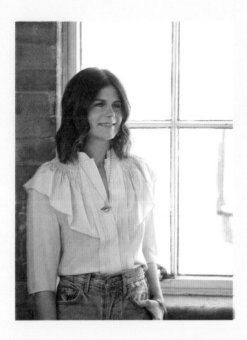

Eve Kalinik BA Hons, Dip NT, mBANT, CNHC, is regarded as one of the most exciting voices in food and health today. Her modern, fresh and innovative approach to gut health, which combines scientific knowledge and practical advice with inspiring and delicious recipes, means that she is in great demand as a nutritional therapist, and as a writer and brand consultant. Aside from her nutritional practice, Eve is a columnist for *Psychologies*, a frequent speaker at various industry events and one of the tutors for *Guardian Masterclasses*.

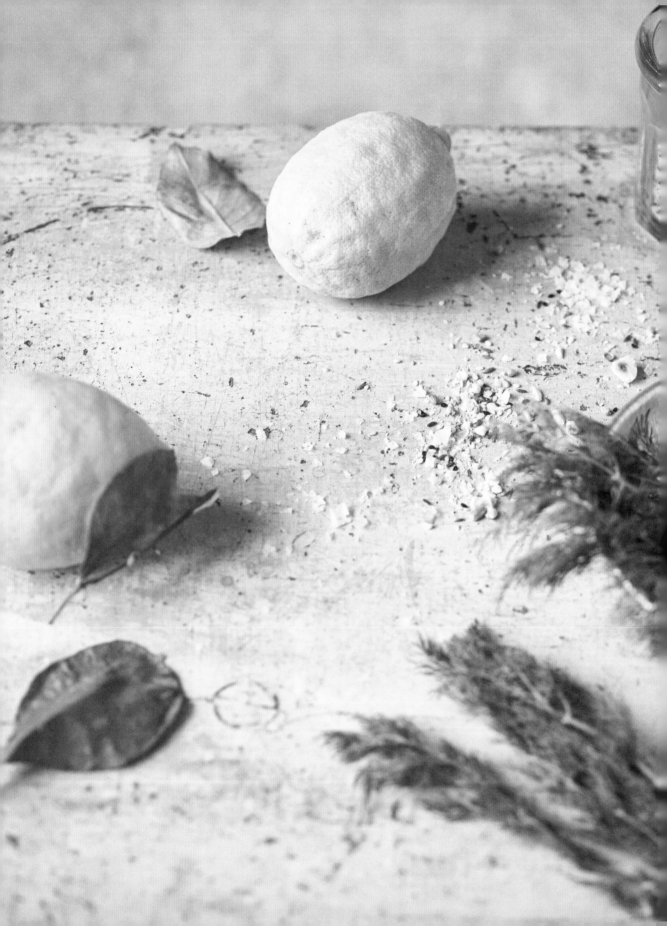

contents

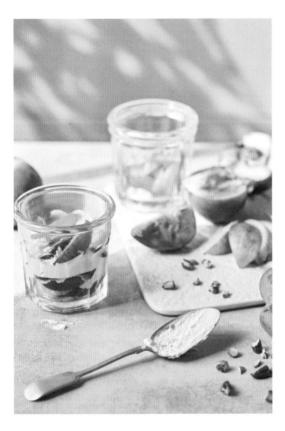
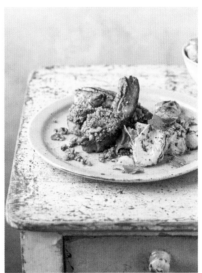
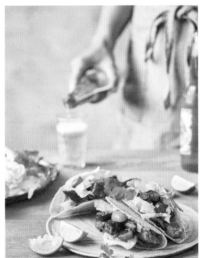

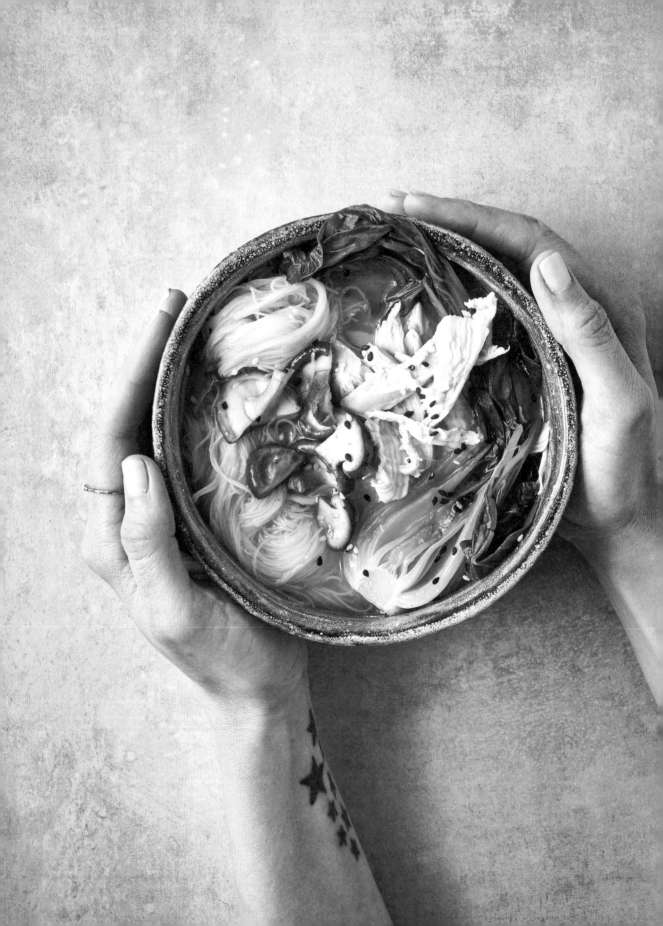

introduction

WE'VE ALL EXPERIENCED those infamous 'gut feelings' that tell us instinctively and intuitively how to respond towards a person, situation or decision. Indeed those feelings are crucial in helping us to better navigate our world and the people in it. However, you might be surprised to know that what may seem like an entirely metaphysical process is, in fact, influenced by some trillions of microbes that live in our gut. This collective of 'mini minds' is called the gut microbiota, and it is increasingly being recognised as playing a vital role in maintaining our mental, as well as our physical, wellbeing.

And recognised it should be! The more we discover about the incredibly important role our gut microbiota has to play in our overall health, the more we can truly appreciate and care for the many microbes that reside within us. However, the reality is that in many ways, we – and notably our gut microbiota and our mind – have suffered the onslaught of our modern lifestyle. The birth and evolution of the digital age has, in a relatively short period, dramatically altered the way we perceive the world and engage with one another and our ability to be present and mindful. Alongside our phones, most of us are also perpetually 'switched on' and this omnipresent and constant connectivity has brought a barrage of unrealistic expectations and insurmountable pressures to our day-to-day existence. It is almost impossible not to be overwhelmed by the sheer pressure and the race to keep up with the constant treadmill of life. And while some aspects of this adrenaline-fuelled lifestyle can be exhilarating, even addictive, physically, our body and mind can't cope. And the potential ramifications of such a fast, furious and unsustainable lifestyle? A clear link with the development of myriad chronic symptoms and diseases, crucially those related to the gut and the mind.

Reconsidering the crucial role of the gut in how we feel both physically and mentally could be a momentous part of helping to support the process of healing the mind.

I can certainly relate to that. Before becoming involved in nutrition and health, my previous career in PR came with a huge amount of pressure, unrealistic deadlines and challenging situations to negotiate. Not surprisingly, after a decade of intense stress I came to the point of total physical and mental burn-out. It wasn't a sudden thing. For years I had overlooked signs that my body wasn't well. Many of the symptoms started with my gut, and over the years they became cumulatively worse and widened into other debilitating issues, such as recurrent infections, fatigue and serious bouts of anxiety and low mood. In an attempt to 'keep on top of my game'

and find some kind of quick 'fix' I took medications and supplements, and spent money on expensive treatments, retreats, healing therapies and such like without really addressing the underlying causes.

At an extremely low point I was forced to take a long and hard look at my life and acknowledge that it was neither sustainable nor fundamentally happy. Something had to change. I started with small changes to my diet, and gradually put an end to the cycle of infections and antibiotics that were impairing my gut, immune system and ultimately my mind. Little by little I began to gain strength and clarity on how to move forward in my life, and it wasn't on that never-ending hamster wheel! Gaining greater clarity and a better state of mind put my gut back on track, and having a healthy gut supported that more thoughtful process. This two-way relationship is a strong, significant and powerful one. I know this first-hand and have worked on supporting this connection with hundreds of clients in my second career as a Nutritional Therapist and Functional Medical Practitioner. Through both my personal and clinical experience it is evident that we cannot support the body, notably the gut, without factoring in how we nourish our mind and vice versa. No amount of good stuff that you put into your gut will mitigate a stressed head and/or a sad state of mind. On the flip side, your mood and mental wellbeing can be influenced by the health and 'happiness' of the trillions of microbes that reside in your gut.

Many clients who come to me with longstanding gut issues tell me that they suffer with co-existing mental and emotional symptoms that are just as debilitating as the physical pains they are experiencing. In fact, I would go so far as to say that *most* clients mention some kind of emotional connection with their gut symptoms, such as anxiety, stress or low mood. We can no longer downplay the connection between the rise of digestive health conditions such as irritable bowel syndrome (IBS) and the simultaneous presentation of symptoms related to the mind. It is becoming pretty evident that the two are intertwined and this is why many scientific studies have focused on, and continue to deepen, our understanding of this bi-directional relationship.

We use many phrases that highlight the gut–brain connection, such as gut-wrenching, gut instinct, gut feeling, but while we intuitively know that there is a real physical connection we may not understand the full complexity of this special bond. What was once thought of as a top down (brain to gut) relationship is actually much more of a partnership. As research becomes more advanced it is highlighting that the gut is not quite as subservient to the brain in our head as we once may have thought. Moreover the gut is not just the 'second' or 'little' brain, as it is often described – but can operate independently of our grey matter.

When you look at the statistics and begin to understand how much the gut microbiome influences our mental health and wellbeing it is truly astounding. For example, 90–95 per cent of the neurotransmitter serotonin, most renowned for its 'happy' effect, is produced and managed in the gut – along with other neurotransmitters, such as dopamine and GABA, that influence how we think and feel. We will delve into this in much more detail throughout the book but it certainly gives some initial food for thought!

how this book can help you

I decided to write this book as an evolution of my first; this time focusing on the powerful gut–brain connection. Having studied psychology at university, mental health and wellbeing has always been an area that is very close to my heart. And knowing now that there is such a close link with the gut, I believe that taking this aspect into account is potentially game-changing for the way we treat mental health and gut-related conditions. Essentially, reconsidering the crucial role of the gut in how we feel both physically and mentally could be a momentous part of helping to support the process of healing the mind.

I begin the book by taking you through the science with easily digestible nuggets of information on how the gut works. This will give you a greater understanding of why, and how, the gut-brain connection is so powerful, as well as some tangible and empowering knowledge to help you improve this relationship.

We will also look at the association between the health of the gut, inflammation and the development of certain mood disorders such as depression, anxiety and stress, as well as cognitive conditions including Parkinson's disease and Alzheimer's. I'll also highlight the importance of sleep and how our gut microbiota can be negatively impacted by not getting decent shut-eye.

Something I'm extremely passionate about is cultivating a better relationship with our food. With that in mind I look at ways of building a more positive connection with the food on our plates. I believe that a healthy and happy relationship with our food, and on a much deeper level with ourselves, relies on an inclusive approach to our diet, rather than restriction and labelling certain foods as 'bad' or 'good'. My goal is to help you gain a more intuitive and mindful approach towards eating and, as a result, a more compassionate and kind attitude to yourself.

Alongside the science you'll find plenty of mind-blowingly tasty recipes. They focus on ingredients that are good for your gut and kind to your mind, but they are not complicated. I've designed them to give you those precious moments of recovery as you enjoy the process of making them and reconnecting with your food, which is one of the main themes of the book. Starting your day with my Bakewell Bircher or Peanut and Miso Muffins, which are brimming with delicious and gut-nourishing ingredients, can bring a positive high to your morning. And in the evening, coming home to my veggie-based Dukkah Cauliflower 'Steak' or simple Harissa Chicken dish will provide a restorative end to your day. These are just some of the delicious recipes that I have lovingly created to feed both belly and soul. If that isn't enough to get your appetite and your attention heightened, you'll also find some wonderful wine pairings with some of the main dishes, if you enjoy the occasional glass with your meal. After all, one of my fundamental principles is that we should celebrate meal times and take time to sit and savour.

You might be reading this book because you simply want to understand the link between the gut and the brain. You may also have gravitated towards it because you, or a friend or family member, are suffering with some kind of mental health, cognitive condition and/or gut-related condition and you want to feel more empowered. Or perhaps, just like me, you are fascinated by the gut and can't get enough of reading about it! Whatever your reason for wanting to know more, this book can help you to better understand how to nourish your mind through supporting your gut.

It is true to say that findings in this area are fairly new. However, the research reveals some very real, exciting and innovative ways to rethink the gut–brain connection. As you read on it will become clear that we need to be mindful of the microbial world that lives within each and every one of us, and just how much of a say our microbes have in both our physical and mental wellbeing. Be in no doubt, the phrase 'trust your gut' will take on an entirely new, significant and powerful meaning by the time you reach the end.

part 1

from top to bottom

PICTURE AN ENTIRE universe with planets and stars, rich, rolling landscapes, scenic diversity, colourful flora and fauna, and trillions of life forms living together in perfect harmony. This might sound like an imaginary galaxy but this extraordinary and unique universe exists in each and every one of us. It is our gut.

For many years the gut was the 'forgotten' organ; however, over the past decade or so it has become a hot topic of conversation and research. And it's thanks to that ongoing scientific research that we have gained significant traction in understanding the intricate workings of the gut and just how much the health of our gut and its trillions of resident microbes affects our physical and mental wellbeing. It transpires that the phrase 'go with your gut' is based on much more than just trusting a hunch.

Before we get into the nitty-gritty of the gut–brain connection it is necessary to have a thorough understanding of what is meant by 'the gut', so, in this opening chapter, I'll set the scene by guiding you through the stages of digestion and the many processes that the gut manages. We will then focus on the trillions of microbes that reside in the gut and why having a healthy gut microbiome is so important for our overall health and wellbeing, including that of the brain. I'll also consider how the gut microbiome establishes itself, right from birth, and the link this has to early brain development.

This chapter will give you a greater understanding – and appreciation – of your truly remarkable gut, and lay the 'groundwork' before we move on to the science behind the gut–brain connection and the practical advice included in the rest of the book.

defining 'the gut'

The gut, aka the gastrointestinal tract, is essentially one long tube that runs from the mouth to the point where our poop exits. As we happily tuck into a meal we don't tend to think about the multitude of complex processes that need to happen for digestion to occur and for us to convert food into fuel.

The workings of the gut are akin to a highly choreographed production that uses hormones to stimulate appetite and muscular movement, activating enzymes to help us break down our food and assimilate and absorb nutrients for our entire body. Our gut is also where the external meets our internal environment. This means that we don't reap the benefits of a meal until it has gone through the lengthy process of digestion and our gut has decided what can, or cannot, pass into our bloodstream.

Not only does our gut have the enormous task of digesting and absorbing nutrients from our food, but it is also responsible for protecting us against anything entering the gut that might cause us harm.

This complex performance simply cannot happen without the assistance of the trillions of microbes in our gut. We'll come to the starring role of those microbes later in the chapter, but it is important to understand that gut health covers the whole process of digestion from start to finish, so let us begin this incredible journey…

for starter

As soon as food enters our mouth we start breaking it down, something that is easily overlooked when we are eating rapidly without much in the way of chewing. Technically called 'mastication', the act of chewing is an important prelude to what happens later on. Chewing stimulates the production of saliva, which contains digestive enzymes that begin the process of dismantling our meal. Consider digestive enzymes to be like chemical grinders that break down our food into smaller molecules so that the gut can assimilate, absorb and process nutrients efficiently. Our saliva contains the digestive enzyme amylase, which is responsible for breaking down carbohydrate starches into sugars: try chewing a piece of bread long enough and it will start to taste sweet – that's amylase kicking in. We also start breaking down dietary fats in the mouth with the assistance of the digestive enzyme lipase. Once our food has been thoroughly chomped, and with the help of saliva initiating the swallowing process, the oesophagus – often called the food pipe or gullet – sends this chewed ball of food, the bolus, on to the next part of the process, the stomach.

Our stomach is essentially our first line of defence, which is why it needs to have a very acidic/low pH environment to kill off any potential pathogens that we may ingest through food or fluid. It maintains this high acidity by releasing gastric juices, primarily hydrochloric acid, from parietal cells that are located in glands in the stomach. Adequate levels of acidity are not only important from a defence perspective but also to ensure that we break down and digest dietary proteins efficiently. This relies on an enzyme called pepsin that is secreted in the stomach and is activated by acidic gastric juices. Our stomach also releases hormones to stimulate the muscles in the gut for motility, as well as those responsible for switching hunger cues on and off. Having been thoroughly churned in the stomach the resulting 'mush', known as chyme, moves on to the next part of its journey, the small intestine.

main course

While it might be called the small intestine, this is actually a misnomer on many levels because what happens here is anything but small. This is where most of digestion and absorption of nutrients from our food takes place. Its sheer size is also misrepresented by its name, since the small intestine is in fact the largest part of the gut. It manages to perform such a sizeable role due to its multi-folded surface that contains tiny finger-like projections, called intestinal villi and microvilli, which sit nicely along the length of the small intestine. These projections are essential for us to absorb the nutrients from our food that are then passed into our bloodstream to support other processes in the body. The structure of the villi means that its surface area is vast, making the small intestine more efficient at absorption. Also embedded in our microvilli are other digestive enzymes called 'brush border' enzymes. These are readily available to help break down sugars and starches such as sucrose and lactase.

However, the small intestine is not solo in its endeavours; crucially it relies on other organs, notably the pancreas, liver and gallbladder, to absorb nutrients from our food. The pancreas is the main site for the production of digestive enzymes in the form of pancreatic juice, which it releases into the small intestine to break down our food further. Alongside this, the liver produces bile, which is almost detergent-like in its actions. Just like washing-up liquid, bile helps to disperse and break down dietary fats into smaller globules so that we can easily absorb them. The liver handily stashes away this bile in the gall bladder, which reacts to hormonal cues to release the bile into the small intestine as and when it is needed.

At this point the remnants of our meal – anything that the small intestine has not absorbed, including dietary fibre – face a gatekeeper in the form of the ileocaecal valve. This checkpoint is important because it means that our small intestine has ample time to get the most out of our meal before giving the green light for it to move on to the last part of its journey.

the sweet finale

The large intestine is where our former meal now finds itself and where the journey gets a bit more relaxed, in that the large intestine likes to take time to move things through. This has a lot to do with our gut microbes because even though they are found throughout the entire gut, the large intestine is their favourite spot to hang out and they need adequate time to heartily enjoy their 'meal'. Remember, the small intestine doesn't care much for dietary fibre, but for our gut microbes these 'leftovers' provide a veritable feast. In return for feeding them fibre, they give back generously by producing substances and messengers that help us to manage inflammation, support the health of the gut barrier, synthesise vitamins, supply mood-influencing neurotransmitters like 'happy' serotonin and also train our immune system so that it knows how to react appropriately. We'll delve into the gut microbiome in more detail in the next section but suffice to say that it is very much a mutualistic relationship.

The culmination of this amazing process is the making of our magical movements – yup, I just called your poop magic! Water is reabsorbed to hydrate the body and the remaining matter forms stools. This is also where our gut collects waste including old red blood cells, gut microbes at the end of their natural life and other toxic by-products that are also part of our poop. All being well this should result in a daily visit to the loo, but it differs from person to person, and there can be many different factors to consider, so don't panic if that's not the case for you. In fact, panicking can throw off the gut–brain connection, which can be part of the issue. So try to make your bathroom trips something to rejoice in, and perhaps take a moment to reflect on the impressive process needed to get to this merry end.

the mighty microbiome

Microbes might be tiny but their effect on our health and wellbeing is something of epic proportions. These trillions of microscopic organisms and their genetic material, which live in and on us, are collectively referred to as the human microbiome, with the largest community existing in the gut. It is important to understand and clarify some of the terminology around this subject as it can be a bit confusing. When we talk about the *microbiome* this refers to microbes *and* their genes and how they communicate/interact with our human cells. The *microbiota* is the term that refers solely to the collective population of microbes themselves. The two are used so interchangeably that if you use one or the other it doesn't really matter, but it is still good to know that they don't mean the exact same thing. I'll be using both terms throughout the book, but whether it is gut microbiota or gut microbiome simply be aware that it refers to all of the trillions of microbes in your gut.

As we happily tuck into a meal we don't tend to think about the multitude of complex processes that need to happen for digestion to occur and for us to convert food into fuel.

The gut microbiota is not made up of bacteria alone, although most of the microbes in the gut are from the bacterial kingdom. Living alongside bacteria are fungi, parasites and viruses, and each of us has our own unique set of gut microbes and genes that make up our personal gut microbiome.

The gut microbiome is prodigious in many ways. What was once put at a ratio of 1:10 in favour of microbes versus human cells in the entire body, is now thought to be closer to 1:1.3. Still, you are technically more microbe than you are human. The other startling fact is that we are 99 per cent microbial from a genetic perspective, as microbes house around 8 million genes, compared to our humbling 23,000.

Microbes also have the advantage of being able to adapt and mutate their genes every 20 minutes, while we have to wait around 10,000 years for evolution to catch up and make such changes happen.

Microbes don't just massively outnumber us in this regard but also in their time on this planet. They have been around a *lot* longer than us. In fact, microbes were the earliest forms of life, first appearing on earth around four billion years ago, and they had the planet to themselves for hundreds of millions of years until the first glimpses of primitive animal life appeared in the form of marine creatures. Microbes found a home in the gut of these sea creatures and in return they helped them to digest food and resist pathogens and toxins. And this beautiful relationship between microbes and their hosts has stood the test of some hundreds of millions of years of evolution and makes the microbiome part of every living being on earth today. Quite simply, if it weren't for microbes we wouldn't be here. This relationship is why there is such a strong connection between us and our tiny comrades.

mutually beneficial

We have a truly symbiotic relationship with our gut microbiota. We provide them with a nice cosy home and a buffet of nutrients, such as dietary fibre and polyphenols (more on these later), and they reciprocate in many positive ways. Let's turn our attention to some of these…

Keeping our natural armour strong

Our gut microbiome teaches and trains our immune system to react appropriately, which starts from the moment we are born. The more exposure that we have to microbes, the more diverse and varied our gut microbiome becomes, which creates an immune system that is better 'educated'. This is, in part, the reason why the development of atopic allergies and auto-immune diseases has been exponentially increasing – we are becoming almost too 'clean' as a result of the overuse of medications like antibiotics, increased elective C-section births and the ubiquitous use of harsh anti-microbial household products. Inadvertently, we are weakening our immune system.

Alongside 'educating' our immune system, our gut microbiome protects us against pathogenic microbes that would otherwise make us ill. Moreover, gut immunity is one of the most important parts of our overall immune system, with the immune cells in gut-associated lymphatic tissue (GALT) accounting for 70–80 per cent of total immune cells in the body.

Synthesising super SCFAs Short-chain fatty acids (SCFAs) are beneficial substances that our gut microbiota generate upon fermenting dietary fibre. SCFAs – specifically butyrate, propionate and acetate – are incredibly important for many processes in the body, including the health of the brain. You'll see butyrate popping up quite a lot throughout the course of the book so it's good to get familiar with it now. Butyrate and the other SCFAs provide energy for the cells that line the gut barrier, helping to keep it strong so that the right things are moving in and out of the gut. We'll look at that and the concept of 'leaky gut' in the next chapter.

SCFAs also help in managing inflammation, communicating with the immune system, stimulating the release of hormones in the gut related to appetite, and supporting motility through the gut – they even contribute to the balance of blood sugar levels in order to keep energy levels stable. Phew, that's quite some list!

Assisting with digestion and absorption
Our gut microbes play a vital role in digesting and helping us absorb nutrients from our food. They produce compounds, such as bile acids and enzymes, that aid the processing and conversion of nutrients. Furthermore, they eat what we can't digest in the form of dietary fibre.

Making vitamins and amino acids Vitamin K, biotin, thiamine, folic acid and B12 are made by gut microbes. The latter of these is vital for cognitive health, and deficiency has been associated with conditions such as depression, anxiety and dementia. Our gut microbes are also able to synthesise amino acids, which are the building blocks of protein so that we have a ready supply if our dietary intake of protein runs low.

Creating and stimulating the release of chemical messengers This includes the action of neurotransmitters such as serotonin, dopamine and GABA, which can exert their influence on emotions and cognitive functioning. Our gut microbiota also has a vital role in producing brain-derived neurotrophic factor (BDNF), crucial for the health of neurons in the brain and something that can be depleted in neuro-degenerative conditions like Parkinson's disease and Alzheimer's. Lower levels of BDNF can also negatively impact our physical ability to handle stress.

Detoxing and metabolising Forget detox diets – together with your liver, the gut microbiota has this covered! Gut microbes help us to detoxify toxins from food and the environment, as well as metabolising medications and hormones such as oestrogen.

Reading through that lengthy list, it becomes clear the sheer amount of work that our gut microbes are doing, and I'm sure you now have a greater appreciation of everything they give back to us and why they are intrinsic to our existence. But how do we achieve such an amicable relationship with them – and maintain it – and what does it actually mean to have a 'healthy balance' of microbes in our gut?

living in harmony

For the most part, we have come to live with microbes in harmonious bliss – after all, it is in both of our interests to have a mutualistic 'you scratch my back, I'll scratch yours' agreement. Co-existing with a healthy and thriving gut microbiota means we reap the rewards of everything it gives back to us and, most of the time, that natural give-and-take relationship works perfectly well.

It is often neither fair nor accurate to assume that a microbe is categorically 'good' or 'bad', as this can often be situation-specific to the environment that the microbe is living in. Just as we might have a bad day and react inappropriately, so can some microbes under particular conditions. For example, this can occur post antibiotic treatment, in certain individuals and/or with those who have weakened immune systems, causing an increase in numbers and heightened 'aggressive' behaviour in microbes that would otherwise reside happily in the gut.

However, for the majority of us this is not a problem because we have our own happy gathering of gut microbes, known as commensal microbes, to counteract any kind of 'inappropriate behaviour'. These are microbes that should be present in our gut and crucially help to maintain a healthy balance in the gut microbiota and keep everything in check.

That said, when the number of potentially 'bad' gut microbes in the gut increase markedly, and the environment is conducive to making them more aggressive, it can unfavourably sway the balance over our own resident commensal 'peacekeepers'. In such instances they have the ability to cause a considerable amount of disruption. When this imbalance occurs in the gut, technically referred to as dysbiosis, it can have a negative effect on all of the processes and systems the gut microbiota helps to manage, including our brain health. Dysbiosis can also create some pretty unpleasant gut symptoms, such as diarrhoea, nausea and inflammation.

Dysbiosis can be the result of factors, usually more than one, including:

- The overuse of certain medications, particularly antibiotics

- Stress and the hormones produced during stress

- A diet lacking in fibre and colour, and one that is high in processed foods and artificial sweeteners (which provide little by way of nourishment for our gut microbes)

- Poor sleep (as our gut microbiota work on a circadian rhythm, just like us, and need some decent shut-eye too)

We'll be looking at all these points in more detail in subsequent chapters. However, it is important to understand that having one, or indeed many, of these factors doesn't necessarily mean that you have dysbiosis. We also have to consider genetics and the gut microbiome we are born with, which leads nicely on to the next section.

born ready

It is truly a collaborative relationship that we have with our microbes, but when it comes to the importance of that relationship nothing is more symbolic than what happens when we are born. This is when we first meet our microbiome. Before we are lovingly cradled in the arms of our mother we are glorified with an almighty welcoming party in the form of trillions of microbes. These 'suitors' are the ones that will lay the foundations for our gut health, and begin to cultivate our immune system and the development of our brain circuitry. As we enter the world through our mother's birth canal, we are literally cocooned in a plethora of microbes passed on from her, and these then start to colonise our gut microbiome – a pivotal moment for setting the scene and determining the future of our gut health.

Microbes might be tiny but their effect on our health and wellbeing is something of epic proportions.

The way in which we are born is therefore of real significance as it defines the beginning and later development of our gut microbiome. Babies born via Caesarean (C-section) are not afforded the same microbial 'fanfare'. Rather than being cocooned with microbes from Mum, the first microbes that they are likely to be exposed to may well be from the skin of the doctors and nurses during delivery, which is not an ideal beginning for the gut microbiome. In fact, it seems that bacteria from the *Bifidobacterium* family take longer to colonise in the gut of a C-section baby than that of a baby born vaginally.

The way in which we inherit our gut microbiome also has a role in helping to shape the wiring of the brain; so much so that C-sections have been linked with a higher prevalence of conditions such as autism (I will come back to that in coming chapters). Of course there are necessary and life-saving reasons for having a Caesarean delivery, but, where it is an elective choice, it might be worth considering giving your baby's biome a head start.

Even before we enter the world it appears our mother's gut microbiota begins to alter: changes begin during the first trimester and continue throughout pregnancy as populations of certain bacteria increase or decline. These changes in the composition of gut microbes could be seen as some kind of natural adaptation to support pregnancy and birth. The other microbial shift happens in the vagina, where *lactobacilli* species increase in numbers in readiness for the baby's birth. This provides a more acidic environment that is less conducive to pathogenic bacteria, thereby providing a safer passage for the baby to enter the world. These *lactobacilli* become the first microbes to populate the baby's gut. They are also the species that help us to break down lactose, the main sugar in breast milk. Nature *is* clever.

Interestingly, it seems that our mother's state of mind during pregnancy can also have a determining role on the gut microbes we inherit. Studies suggest that stress during pregnancy can shift the balance of the vaginal microbiome towards one that contains fewer *lactobacilli* species. Stress management during pregnancy is therefore an important part of nourishing the health of Mum's gut microbiome, so that she can pass on a richer set of microbes to her offspring. And, of course, nourish her own mental wellbeing too!

baby biome and brain

Beyond birth and into breastfeeding, the milk from our mother is unique in complexity in that it contains bacteria to feed microbes in our gut. Equally, our gut microbes help us to digest some of the sugars contained in breast milk, which we would otherwise struggle to break down and absorb. Breast milk also contains essential fatty acids that help to support the composition of the gut microbiota, as well as being a significant nutrient for brain development. It is another example of the co-evolution between us and our tiny yet mighty microbes.

While a baby may not formulate its first words for several years, the 'chatter' between the gut microbiome and the brain is a 'conversation' that has already started. As we have just explored, the way we are born is a key factor in the foundation of our gut microbiome. Another relates to our mother's milk. Our gut microbes are perfectly primed to metabolise the milk sugars and complex carbohydrates in breast milk: babies cannot digest these carbohydrates but, guess what, microbes can! In fact, this is perfect 'food' for the bacteria *Bifidobacterium infantis,* a key starter species in the making of the gut microbiome, along with other compounds in breast milk that also favour the growth of beneficial bacteria.

Mothers also pass on crucial antibodies in colostrum: these are important for the development of the immune system, which is a key communication channel to the brain. Furthermore, breast milk contains fatty acids that nourish the growth of neurons (nerve cells) and the gut microbiome itself. Nature designed breast milk to support the baby and the cultivation of a healthy and thriving gut microbiome, and that ultimately leads to a stronger and more resilient constitution for us. It is truly magical. However, breastfeeding isn't an option for every mother and it can be fraught with difficult emotions. In this case it is best to focus attention on strengthening the bond between mother and child, rather than getting overly anxious. After all, breast milk is only one of many factors that contribute to nourishing the early development of our gut microbiome.

As we grow, our gut microbiota extends in number as well as developing in complexity and diversity. The first three years are a crucial period for our gut microbiome, as it is the most dynamic transition phase. Its development comes predominantly from the food we eat and is very much reliant on the intake of varied sources of dietary fibre to support a more heterogenous and healthier gut. Our exposures to people and places can also contribute to the ever-developing rolling landscape of our gut

microbiome. Children who grow up in rural locations, for example, tend to accumulate more in the way of microbial diversity, being that they are generally more exposed to bacteria than those raised in urban environments. For each of us these exposures will be different and make up what is our unique gut microbiome.

Alongside 'educating' our immune system, our gut microbiome protects us against pathogenic microbes that would otherwise make us ill

In the next chapter we will explore the fascinating and enlightening 'conversation' between our 'little' gut brain and the brain in our head, which impacts how we feel physically *and* emotionally. It is truly mind-blowing.

brain and the bugs

IT IS HIGHLY likely that you will have experienced that 'fluttery' feeling deep in your gut, commonly described by the idiom 'butterflies in the stomach'. It is one of our natural instincts in anticipation of something we find challenging, nerve-wracking or even exhilarating.

You may have encountered this sensation in situations such as delivering a big presentation, preparing to sit an exam or as part of first-date nerves. This is the physical reaction when we are faced with something that causes us some level of trepidation or heightened anxiety.

You might therefore think that this is purely an emotionally driven and brain-dependent 'gut feeling', but there is a much deeper and meaningful connection to our gut; one that affects how we think, feel and even behave.

It is our gut microbiota, as it has a momentous and highly influential role in how our brain operates. So, rather than imagining butterflies in the stomach, it is much more accurate to contemplate the colossal numbers of microbes in the gut. When we talk about the gut–brain connection, we really need to think about it as more of a menáge-à-trois between the microbiota, gut and the brain. This is what we will explore further throughout this chapter.

smarty pants

When we think about the foundations of our mental health, including thoughts, feelings and behaviour, the first organ that naturally springs to mind is the brain. But the mind-blowing thing is that we have two brains. Yup you guessed it. I'm talking about the gut – our 'second' (or 'little') brain, a phrase coined by Michael Gershon in his 1998 book *The Second Brain*. Just as the brain contains billions of communicating nerve cells known as neurons, the gut also houses a sizeable 500 million neurons, and communicates to the rest of the body in similar ways. Suffice to say this 'gut chat' relies very much on the gut microbiota and puts a whole new spin on the phrase smarty pants.

Let's start by looking at the nervous system that makes up our second brain and how this interacts with the one in our head.

gut ground control

The enteric nervous system (ENS) is the main way in which your gut 'thinks'; it consists of a highly intricate network of nerves embedded in the tissue lining the gut. Think of it as the ground control system for the gut. The ENS is part of the peripheral nervous system (PNS): the part of the nervous system outside the central nervous system (CNS) – the brain and spinal cord. The PNS has two divisions: the somatic nervous system, which governs voluntary movements, such as jumping up and down or riding a bike (basically stuff that your brain tells your body to do), and the autonomic nervous system (ANS), which manages involuntary processes such as breathing and digestion (things we don't have to think about doing). The ENS is usually considered to be a branch of the ANS because, other than chewing, we don't have to activate the process of digestion.

The ENS contains the most complex of 'nerve circuits' outside the central nervous system (CNS) and it houses somewhere in the region of 200–600 million neurons – more than the spinal cord. These nerve circuits consist of masses of nerve tissue, called ganglia, which are embedded in the walls of the gut, including the stomach, small intestine and colon, as well as the pancreas. Within the ENS exists various sensory and motor neurons that influence gut functions, including peristalsis (the wave-like muscular motion of the gut), communicating to cells in the barrier of the gut to allow substances in and out, and stimulating the parietal cells in the stomach to produce hydrochloric acid. Having its own nervous system means that the ENS is the *only* organ that can operate independently of the CNS hence 'the second or little brain'.

gut–brain speak

Now that you have a basic understanding of the ENS and the intricate workings of the gut's nervous system, we can start to explore the bi-directional communication in the gut–brain axis, which should really be referred to as the microbiota–gut–brain axis.

There are three main pathways that our microbes, gut and brain use to 'speak' to one another so let's look at each of these.

speed dial

The first of these is the nerve pathway and it is the most direct, via the ENS and central nervous system, and uses chemical messengers called neurotransmitters. The microbiota makes, manages and communicates using the same neurotransmitters as the brain. This is a crucial point: the same neurotransmitters that govern different physical processes, as well as emotional feelings in the body, occur in the gut as well as the brain. As such these neurotransmitters, as well as other substances produced by our gut microbiota such as SCFAs, can have a significant influence on both our physical and mental health and wellbeing. We will look at these in more detail shortly; for now you simply need to bear in mind that neurotransmitters are the main language used in this type of microbiota–gut–brain communication.

The microbiota makes, manages and communicates using the same neurotransmitters as the brain. This is a crucial point.

The main channel for this type of communication between the gut and the brain is the vagus nerve, which is part of the autonomic nervous system (ANS). The name derives from the Latin for 'wandering' and reflects the way the nerve meanders from the brain to the lowest part of the abdomen, touching on other organs on its way. (This includes the diaphragm, which is why diaphragmatic breathing is so helpful for the gut and managing stress). This direct channel allows the brain to send signals to the gut, and vice versa, with speed and efficiency. This is vitally important so that the brain can quickly be alerted should the gut deem that something requires urgent attention. If you remember from the first chapter the gut is privy to a lot of information and responsibility that can compromise our wellbeing – it primarily has to manage where the external meets our internal. The brain needs to know ASAP if something has gone awry or amiss.

A prime example of this is the typical 'fight or flight' stress response versus 'rest and digest' opposing response. In activating the 'fight or flight' mode the ENS gut–brain's response is to slow down or halt digestion altogether. Think of the expression 'frozen with fear' and you get the gist of what happens in the gut too. This process occurs to allow all our energy to be geared towards the imminent danger. When we switch into fight or flight mode all systems, other than those helpful to our immediate survival, become much less of a priority. This is why chronic stress can be so debilitating. On the other end of the vagus nerve line, our gut microbiota can reciprocate and communicate back to the brain using some of the same types of neurotransmitter language to signal their own alarm bells should it be required.

immune alert

Another way that the microbiota–gut–brain axis communicates is via the immune system. Remember that our gut manages the barrier between the external and the internal to control what can be passed into the body and what needs to be eliminated. It is the site for the greater proportion of our immune system so it is important that potential threats are communicated effectively to the brain.

A healthy gut microbiota regulates this immune response by reacting to anything that might disrupt the general 'status quo' in the body. The gut microbiota prompts immune cells (immunocytes) to mount an anti- or pro-inflammatory response using small proteins called cytokines to elicit the appropriate reaction from other immune cells. These signals stimulate nerve cells in the gut and are then sent to the brain via the vagus nerve to communicate the degree of inflammation. Both the gut microbiota and the cells that line the gut can produce these cytokine chemicals.

This is all well and good with a healthy gut microbiota, because it stimulates the appropriate chain of responses from our immune system. However, if we have a compromised gut microbiota, the wrong prompts can be sent. This creates confusion with the responses and surveillance from immune cells and may lead to chronic and systemic inflammation, including the brain – which is why inflammation has been implicated in the development of certain mental health and cognitive conditions.

Conversely, chronic mental stress impairs the way that the immune system responds: if we are constantly in 'fight or flight' mode our body's main focus is on survival. Moreover, the hormones that are produced during stress can have a negative impact on the health of the microbiota and the gut barrier, which means that immune responses are more likely to be skewed and the gut barrier can be breached, with substances moving or 'leaking' into the bloodstream that should be kept within the gut. (We will look in more detail at 'leaky gut' in the next chapter.)

the HPA way

The third pathway for microbiota–gut–brain 'chat' is a lot subtler and involves the endocrine system, the network of glands that secrete hormones. The hypothalamus is the area of the brain that links the central nervous system with the endocrine system and it plays a vital role in ANS activity. The pituitary gland is the most notable endocrine gland and is responsible for maintaining the body's overall internal balance, or homeostasis, through hormones. The hypothalamus, pituitary gland and peripheral endocrine glands together make up the neuroendocrine system.

The main pathway for all this communication is via the hypothalamus–pituitary–adrenal (HPA) axis. Gut microbes are crucial to the development and function of this axis so if the gut microbiota have been compromised it can induce an exaggerated HPA stress response. This imbalance can be caused by stress hormones such as cortisol and medications like antibiotics, which have a negative impact on the composition of our gut microbiota. Furthermore, if our immune system is sending out lots of pro-inflammatory messages to the brain, as mentioned earlier, this can also trigger the stress response in the HPA axis and it can become a bit of an inflammatory-stress loop. (We will look at stress in much more detail in Chapter 4.)

Besides the HPA stress response, gut microbes also have an effect on other endocrine glands, and their communication to the brain, by helping to regulate hormones. This includes detoxifying oestrogen and converting thyroid hormones into their more active form. In addition, the gut microbiota has a role in managing the release of hormones such as insulin, glucagon, gastrin and leptin that feed back to the brain in order to control appetite signals and blood sugar levels.

happy talk

Now that we have examined the main channels of microbiota–gut–brain communication let's look at neurotransmitters, the chemical messengers that your nerve cells use to communicate with one another. Neurotransmitters are produced in our brain and secreted and managed by our gut microbiome. They are the main 'language' used in the microbiota–gut–brain nerve pathway, so let's look at some of them in more detail…

serotonin

Serotonin, famously dubbed the 'happy' neurotransmitter, plays a major part in mood and cognition. However, you may be pretty astonished to know that a whopping 90–95 per cent of serotonin is produced in the gut. Serotonin is made from the amino acid tryptophan, which is converted into 5-hydroxytryptamine (5-HT), aka serotonin. We need to take in tryptophan through our diet, and it can be found in a wide variety of protein-rich foods, such as turkey, chicken, eggs, oily fish, peanuts and pumpkin seeds.

Gut microbiota directly and indirectly influence serotonin levels. The vast majority of serotonin production in the gut depends on special endocrine cells called enterochromaffin cells (ECs) that sit in the lining of the gut and are packed full of this happy neurotransmitter. Microbes in our gut produce substances, including short-chain fatty acids like butyrate, that essentially 'switch on' these cells to

release serotonin. It is a team effort between microbes and the ECs. In addition to this, our gut microbiota can directly synthesise serotonin and, while this peripheral serotonin cannot cross the blood–brain barrier (BBB), our gut microbes control the availability of the precursor amino acid tryptophan, which does cross the BBB and is converted into serotonin in the brain.

dopamine

Just as our gut microbiota can directly synthesise serotonin, it can make other neurotransmitters, such as dopamine, that are used peripherally in the body. In fact, 50 per cent of overall dopamine is synthesised in the gut. In the brain, dopamine is associated with pleasure and the reward system; in the gut, it helps to coordinate the contraction of muscles in the colon. Like gut-derived serotonin, it is believed that peripheral dopamine is not able cross the BBB. However, our gut microbes can influence the amount of tyrosine available, which does cross the BBB and is the precursor amino acid used to make dopamine in the brain. Tyrosine is found in protein-rich foods such as chicken, fish, yogurt, sesame seeds and also avocado and bananas. When we consider that at least half of dopamine is produced in the gut it again emphasizes the role that our gut microbiota can play in supporting the health of our brain.

GABA

Another neurotransmitter produced by our gut microbiota is GABA (gamma-amino butyric acid). GABA is the body's major inhibitory neurotransmitter, which means that it reduces over-activity of neurons in the brain and the central nervous system. It does this by binding itself to nerve cell receptors, hindering their ability to receive and send messages to other neurons. This is very important as too many neuronal signals can result in conditions such as seizures and epilepsy, and has also been linked to mood disorders. While it was thought that GABA cannot cross the BBB, current research is suggesting that it may be able to do so in small amounts.

GABA production can be boosted by eating foods that are rich in its precursor, glutamate. These include oats, walnuts, lentils and green and black tea – tea is also high in l-theanine, which additionally increases GABA levels. Fermented foods are also high in glutamate and since they also contain beneficial bacteria that can produce their own supply of GABA, eating fermented foods could have a double whammy GABA boost!

positive return

Another way our gut microbiota communicates with our brain is via neuroactive substances that it produces. These are called SCFAs (short–chain fatty acids) such as butyrate, propionate and acetate, which we looked at briefly in Chapter 1. Our gut microbiota is able to generate SCFAs upon fermenting dietary fibre. Collectively these fatty acids help with managing inflammation, supporting the immune system and affecting the overall health of the brain. SCFAs are recognised by cells lining the gut that have a crucial role in managing our immune system, and they can therefore have an impact on both the nervous and the immune systems. Furthermore, they can cross the BBB to regulate neurotransmitter synthesis and brain development.

The most widely researched SCFA is butyrate. As well as playing a role in managing inflammation throughout the body, it provides an energy source for the cells that line the gut, maintaining the integrity of the gut barrier and allowing the correct substances to pass through into the bloodstream. It is also believed that, in a similar way to maintaining a robust gut barrier, butyrate helps to manage the integrity of the BBB. Butyrate is almost exclusively made by gut microbes, therefore we rely on a healthy and thriving gut microbiota in order to produce sufficient amounts. If this falls short then it can compromise the intestinal barrier and potentially allow pro–inflammatory chemicals, such as lipopolysaccharides (LPS) and cytokines, to move into the bloodstream rather than being kept within the safe confines of the gut. This breach of the gut barrier is often referred to as intestinal permeability, or 'leaky gut'.

It makes evolutionary sense that our gut microbes might have an influence over the foods that we eat.

Furthermore, when these pro-inflammatory substances 'leak out' there is the potential for a much wider inflammatory effect, and elevated levels of these chemicals have been found in people with certain neurological conditions. It therefore seems logical to consider that a leaky gut can negatively affect the health of the brain.

There is also some evidence that propionate, another SCFA, along with other hormones in the gut, can influence appetite, which could go some way to explaining why we might crave fast-release carbohydrates and sugar. Is it really our gut microbes craving cake? Actually, that's not such a far-fetched concept. It makes evolutionary sense that our gut microbes might have an influence over the foods that we eat, as it is in their interest to be served up their favourite dishes. It isn't implausible to suggest that your cravings may be driven, at least in part, by your gut microbiota and not just your mind. Let's look at that now...

what's driving your hunger?

On a fundamental level the food we eat depends on physical hunger and appetite signals, where we live, availability and cost. Then there are the food choices we make that are driven largely by taste, preference, cultural and potentially ethical reasons – as well as the images and latest diet fads we are continually bombarded with through our daily newsfeed or social media channels. Clearly there are many factors that influence our relationship with food, but few of us consider the important role that our gut microbiota plays in this complex mix.

hungry bugs

Let's begin by looking at the specific hormones that drive and diminish our hunger. These hormones act on the hypothalamus, an area of the brain that oversees our daily intake of food and our eating behaviour. The hypothalamus has been finely tuned by evolution to govern the appropriate amount of energy we need to take in through our food. It constantly assesses our requirements and regulates our metabolism using the extensive input it receives from hormones.

Ghrelin is our 'hunger hormone'. When your stomach is empty, cells located in its lining secrete ghrelin, which is sent to the hypothalamus to signal that it is time to eat. The stomach also seems to release ghrelin in response to bitter flavours being ingested, which is interesting when you think of the bitter-tasting aperitifs that are traditionally offered in Italy and Scandinavia, for example, as a way of preparing your gut for the food to come. At the end of a meal, when we are nicely satisfied, our gut releases appetite-suppressing hormones such as leptin and peptide YY (PYY). This switches off the need to eat so that we know when enough is enough. This is broadly how it has worked for millennia. However, in more recent years it seems as though there might be some 'glitches' in this appetite system which could help further our understanding of the issues around weight management and even obesity.

One reason that has been suggested for this glitch is low-grade and chronic inflammation, which can disrupt microbiota–gut–brain communication. Over time, this can trigger the release of pro-inflammatory substances – like the cytokines mentioned earlier – that may damage the lining of the gut and lead to a more permeable gut barrier.

As the gut barrier becomes more and more breached inflammatory substances can cross the gut barrier and activate a pro-inflammatory immune response, resulting in an overall state of inflammation in the body. This systemic inflammation can interfere with an appropriate response to leptin so that the brain doesn't receive cues that we have had enough to eat, hence we don't receive the appropriate signal to stop. It has been suggested that this disjointed and inflammatory feedback loop can lead to overeating and weight gain, and is why obesity is often referred to as a disease of inflammation. Further to this the increased systemic presence of pro-inflammatory cytokines can interfere with insulin response which can result in increased storage of fat, especially around the abdominal area.

your bugs have cravings too

Many people experience food cravings, and compulsive eating and food addiction are very real. Part of this could be due to the muddled communication between the gut and brain outlined above, but another issue relates to the dopamine reward system. Dopamine is one of the so-called 'feel-good' neurotransmitters outlined earlier, and is associated with the reward system that gives us a sense of pleasure – it is this that is activated in addictive behaviours.

How much influence do we really have over our food choices? Could you be harbouring 'greedy' microbes?

The dopamine reward system is also hooked up to our appetite regulation hormones, so it can be switched on or off on the command of some of the same hormones that work on the hypothalamus. This makes sense in terms of evolution: when calorie-dense, high-fat and high-sugar foods were scarce our hormones motivated us to find these foods and rewarded us with a feeling of pleasure when we ate them. However, in our modern society, where these foods are available at any time, it is all too easy to end up overconsuming, with a 'reward'

feedback to encourage us to seek out these 'feel-good' foods. Chuck in the barrage of advertising to compound the problem and it's easy to see how temptation can get the better of us. We essentially become conditioned to keep eating high-sugar, high-fat foods.

Furthermore, because our gut microbes produce and influence dopamine, it has been suggested that they may have some ability to sway our dopamine reward system towards specific foods *they* have a preference for eating. This makes sense for their own survival and to give them a superior positioning in the gut over other microbes. It also raises the question of how much of an influence we really have over our food choices? Could we be harbouring 'greedy' microbes? This might not be as incomprehensible as it seems, and whilst it would be entirely misleading to label specific microbes as having the ability to influence a leaner physique there does seem to be correlations with certain compositions of the overall gut microbiota profile. Studies have demonstrated that a higher proportion of the firmicutes group of bacteria than bacteroidetes bacteria were associated with increased inflammation and obesity. There is the tongue-in-cheek comment 'Firmicutes make you fat' but the reality is that these gut bacteria are particularly adept at extracting energy (calories) from food, useful when food was scarce, but which means increased caloric absorption and the risk of weight gain when food is so readily available and calorie-dense. In contrast, the studies found that gut microbiota profiles with a higher proportion of bacteroidetes bacteria and a generally more diverse population of microbes were associated with a naturally leaner physique.

Two other bacteria identified in gut microbiota profiling that have also been linked with a leaner body weight include *Akkermansia muciniphila* and *Christensenella minuta*. *Akkermansia* helps to promote mucus production that strengthens the gut barrier, which is important to consider when a compromised or 'leaky' gut barrier can correlate with obesity. In addition, *Akkermansia* produce the SCFA acetate which has a role to play in appetite and regulating the storage of body fat. Levels may be increased through increasing prebiotic foods (see page 62 for more on this). However *Christensenella* seems to be largely down to a genetic lottery, meaning that it is more likely that this bacterium will reside in the gut if it has been inherited.

Given all of this, it doesn't seem unrealistic to speculate that weight management might have much less to do with willpower than many people believe, and it certainly questions the basic 'calories in versus calories out' theory. In fact, could our weight and our penchant for specific foods have some very significant correlations with the bugs in our gut? These are cutting-edge and somewhat controversial opinions but they do certainly provide food for thought.

psychobiotics

Psychobiotics refers to supporting the health of the gut microbiota and using probiotic supplementation to directly target and positively enhance brain function. It's an innovative and ground-breaking new area in the field of neuroscience, pioneered by Irish scientists Professor Ted Dinan and Professor John Cryan at University College Cork.

They researched how the food we eat affects the gut microbiota, and how gut microbes can in turn influence our emotions. The suggestion is that beneficial bacteria ingested from probiotic supplements or fermented foods have the potential to change the output of neurotransmitters and ultimately shape the health of our brain. This could have a major impact on conditions related to cognitive health. Where this gets even more exciting is the potential to target the microbiome using probiotic therapy to treat depression and other psychiatric illness.

Their research indicates that certain microbes have a tendency to supply us with a given neurotransmitter. For instance, lactobacillus bacteria produce more GABA (gamma-amino butyric acid), which has a calming effect, enterococcus strains seem to have a penchant for giving us 'happy' serotonin, while bacillus affords us dopamine for movement, motivation and pleasure. Since evidence of psychobiotic-induced cognitive enhancements in humans is limited and a great deal more research is required, it is very important not to change or stop any medications without the guidance of your GP. It is inspiring, though, to consider a future where we might be able to use prescriptive probiotic treatment to target cognitive conditions. Now that would be smart stuff.

tiny yet mighty minds

As you will have gathered from this chapter, the link between our microbiota, gut and brain depends on their working and communicating together as a trio for the greater good. Our gut microbes can interact with our brain in many ways, and it's clear just how much the microbiota and its trillions of microbial 'minds' uses its very own intelligence system to influence our thoughts, feelings and behaviour.

There's no doubt that having a rich and thriving gut microbiome supports a more positive outlook for the health of our body and our brain. We crucially rely on all these forms of communication from our gut microbes for both our physical and mental wellbeing. It seems that a well-nourished gut microbiome supports a well-nourished mind.

This knowledge might lead us to totally reconsider what 'gut intuition' really means, and perhaps to better trust that innate instinct, knowing that our gut bugs have a sizeable impact on how we think and feel. In many regards they are the ones in the driving seat. I rather like a quote from Professor John Cryan: 'If microbes are controlling the brain, then microbes are controlling everything.'

3

mood, mind and microbes

WOULD IT SOUND completely outrageous if I told you that some of your darkest moments of despair, as well as those of sheer joy, could be influenced by the trillions of tiny microbes living in your gut? You may find the concept incomprehensible, but the striking reality is that our moods and cognitive functioning can be affected by the health of our gut microbiome.

In this chapter we will be exploring the significant effect that our gut microbiome has on the way we feel, think and behave, and the link to conditions such as mood

disorders, neurodegenerative conditions and autism. When we look at mental health conditions and their link with gut health the one key common denominator throughout is inflammation, so this will be a key focus in this chapter. We will be examining the effects of a gut microbiome that is 'mismanaging' the process of inflammation and how this can affect the health of our brain. Further to this, I will highlight some of the crucial substances produced by our gut microbiota that provide 'food' for mood and mind. Inflammation is also a challenge to the health of the gut microbiome as we age, so I'll conclude the chapter with a look at how we can best support our trillions of tiny comrades as we progress into our later years.

Happiness, it seems, is not just a state of mind but one of microbial temperament too. You, and the brain in your head, might be quite happily bobbing along and, if all is well with the 'little brain' in your gut, you can be blissfully unaware of the relationship between the two. But when things go awry, it's a different matter.

the inflamed brain

The microbiota–gut–brain connection has become a huge area of discussion and research, with potentially revolutionary clinical findings now suggesting that it plays a crucial role in managing inflammation; and that inflammation itself could be a significant factor in the development of certain cognitive conditions.

Anyone who has suffered or has been close to someone suffering from depression is familiar with the feeling of being in the depths of despair, engulfed by dark and catastrophic thoughts, as though the brain is literally 'on fire'. And we now know that inflammation may play a significant part in the development of this debilitating condition. Similarly, studies indicate that children with autism show elevated levels of pro-inflammatory chemicals, such as lipopolysaccharides (which form part of the cell wall of certain bacteria), as well as other substances linked to a more permeable gut, including propionic acid (PPA), which suggests some kind of breach in the gut barrier and, as a result, heightened inflammation.

It seems then that inflammation, which is intrinsically related to the health of the gut and gut microbiota, is implicated in many cognitive conditions. Here's how…

leaky gut

In the previous chapter we learned how the gut and brain communicate via the immune system. When this system is compromised it can create a cascade of inflammatory processes that can have ramifications for our overall health, including that of our brain. Essentially, having a healthy gut and gut microbiota means that one of the most important processes that takes place in the gut – that of allowing substances that should be moving in and out of the gut to pass through without hassle, while blocking those that should be kept within the confines of the gut – runs smoothly. However, when the gut barrier is damaged or neglected, due to a shift in the composition of the gut microbiota, stress, poor diet and/or our immune system being under so much duress that it has to focus on the most immediate and pressing demands, this can result in a more permeable or 'leaky' gut. This means that potentially pathogenic bacteria, lipopolysaccharides and even proteins from food can sneak out of the gut and run amok. Unsurprisingly, this creates havoc for our immune system and starts ringing all sorts of inflammatory bells, resulting in the excessive secretion of cytokines, those tiny pro-inflammatory molecules I mentioned in the previous chapter.

As more and more of these substances 'leak' out of the gut, it can set off an inflammatory process that spreads throughout the entire body – akin to lighting a wildfire that can be driven by the health of the gut and the gut microbiota. Ultimately this leaves the body in a state of chronic low-grade inflammation, which can have a negative impact on the brain. As well as being implicated in the development of mood disorders such depression and anxiety, as mentioned earlier, increased permeability of the gut, alongside imbalances in the gut microbiota, have been associated with a higher prevalence towards developing other neurological conditions, including Alzheimer's, Parkinson's disease and autism.

strength in numbers and diversity

Another thing to bear in mind when we are looking at factors that may influence inflammation in the gut–brain connection is the composition, diversity and abundance of our gut microbiota. A rich and varied collection of microbes generally equals a much healthier, stronger and happier gut. Reduced diversity in the gut microbiome and dysbiosis (the imbalance of 'good' and 'bad' bacteria) appear to correlate with cognitive conditions such as mood disorders. Children with autism also often simultaneously have digestive symptoms – like abdominal pain, bloating and constipation, as well as alterations in the composition of the gut microbiota itself – that are different from children without autism. As we have already seen, the colonisation of microbes in our gut not only lays the foundations for gut and immune health, it fundamentally helps to shape the circuits in our brain. In fact, C-section delivery and early childhood antibiotic use have been linked to autism so the gut microbiota is one factor to consider in this picture.

A varied and thriving gut microbiota funda- mentally relies on the food that we give to our gut microbes, which we will look at more in Chapter 6. Essentially, though, if we don't provide adequate amounts and diverse sources of dietary fibre, amongst other key nutrients, this can eventually lead to an undernourished gut microbiota that has a reduced propensity to manage inflammation. It seems that the more heterogenous our gut microbiota, the better we are at retaining a calmer situation in the body and brain.

microbes and mitochondria

When considering what may contribute to an inflamed microbiota–gut–brain connection, we also need to look at the role of mitochondria, the energy powerhouses that exist in almost every single one of our cells. Mitochondria are responsible for generating ATP (adenosine triphosphate), which is the prime source of fuel for cells to function. Mitochondria are believed to have originated from bacteria and, just like our gut microbiota, have their own genetic material. Moreover, since mitochondria are of bacterial origin, they react to substances and signals produced and prompted by our gut microbiota, such as butyrate and inflammatory cytokines, as mentioned in the previous chapter. Therefore, if we have a compromised gut microbiota that is sending off inappropriate signals it can impair the function of the mitochondria.

Both mitochondria and the gut microbiota play a crucial role in the process of apoptosis, which essentially means 'cell suicide', or programmed cell death. It is important for this to happen so that we can terminate unhealthy cells and allow space for new, healthy cells to grow. Apoptosis

the gluten conundrum

One controversial factor in the debate over the causes of 'leaky gut' is the potential role of food allergies and intolerances. In particular, there seems to be a lot of attention given to gluten as a possible contributing factor.

Before we delve into this deeper, we need to differentiate between coeliac disease and gluten sensitivity. Coeliac disease refers to an allergy to gluten, the main protein in wheat products. For those suffering with coeliac disease, eating even the tiniest amount of gluten will elicit an immune-mediated response that destroys the villi that line the gut, thereby affecting overall absorption of nutrients. Unfortunately, gluten is almost everywhere, including in most types of bread, pasta, noodles, cookies, cakes, biscuits, crackers, and even in soy sauce and other condiments. Irrespective of the amount of gluten, the immune system essentially perceives it as a danger or threat. Coeliac disease can be diagnosed via a blood test and/or biopsy.

Gluten sensitivity, on the other hand, wouldn't present with the same blood antibodies but someone may feel that their symptoms improve when they remove foods containing gluten from their diet. This is a bit of a grey area as it can be the case that people test negative for coeliac disease, even though the pattern of symptoms fits with that diagnosis. With some cognitive conditions, such as autism, there have been reported improvements in symptoms when gluten is removed from the diet, but we also have to consider other contributing factors that may have led to the point where the immune system is essentially confused. One has to look at the overall health of the gut microbiome, as we know that it is our gut microbes that essentially give our immune system guidance.

We therefore need to consider factors that may have compromised the gut microbiota; for example, a diet low in dietary fibre, high levels of stress, C-section birth and exposure to antibiotics, especially during infancy. These can all affect the health of the gut microbiota and our immune system, which can lead to an increased predisposition for food sensitivities, including gluten. We have to ask the question, *Is it just as much about nourishing and supporting the health of the gut microbiome, as it is about simply removing food groups?* In the case of gluten sensitivity, it could be that a combination of the two is needed, in order to allow the immune system and the gut microbiome to essentially 'reset'. Let's be clear: we are talking about sensitivities here and not allergies. If you are diagnosed with coeliac disease then you must entirely avoid gluten, although that doesn't mean to say that you can't give some undivided attention to your gut microbiome.

can go 'wrong', however, when the functioning of the mitochondria and gut microbiota are compromised since both have such a directional role in this process. As such, the recognition of healthy versus non-healthy cells gets mixed up and our immune system can attack perfectly healthy cells.

Indeed, this confusion is thought to be one of the key underlying mechanisms that can lead to the destruction of neurons in neurodegenerative conditions, such as Alzheimer's and Parkinson's, and is also believed to be linked to the overall decline in our cognitive functioning as the years go by. Nourishing the health of the gut and the gut microbiota can therefore support our mitochondria to fire on all cylinders and help to temper the flames of inflammation. And although the old saying is if you can't stand the heat get out of the kitchen, that's actually where you want to be heading to boost those good bugs in your gut.

brain 'food'

The health of the microbiota–gut–brain connection depends on our gut microbes providing us with a regular supply of substances that essentially 'feed' our mind and mood. Let's look at some of them now…

butyrate

The production of butyrate, a vital short-chain fatty acid (SCFA), by our gut microbiota is one of the ways that our gut helps to positively manage inflammation in the entire body, including the brain. Studies indicate that lower levels of butyrate are associated with an increased prevalence of mood disorders and neurodegenerative conditions. This

makes sense because butyrate has a key role in regulating our immune system and has a systemic anti-inflammatory effect in the body. Crucially, it is needed as the main energy source for the cells that line the barrier of the gut and if the gut lining is weakened it can result in 'leaky gut' that, as mentioned previously, can have an effect on the health of our brain. Butyrate is also important for the health and integrity of the blood–brain barrier. Further to this, butyrate can enter the brain, acting as an antidepressant in itself and it also suppresses the activity of immune cells and proteins like cytokines that drive inflammation.

The microbiota requires dietary fibre to produce butyrate so, if we are not providing it with enough of its favourite energy source, it will not produce sufficient amounts of the stuff. I'll outline what to eat to boost the gut microbiota and the production of butyrate in Chapter 6.

BDNF

Our gut microbiota has a critical role in the production of brain-derived neurotrophic factor (BDNF), a protein that supports the health and growth of neurons and overall cognitive function. It has been found to be decreased in the brains and blood of patients with anxiety and Alzheimer's, correlating with a compromised gut microbiome.

It is therefore a significant factor to consider in the development of neurodegenerative conditions. Butyrate helps to increase BDNF, so nourishing a healthy balance of microbes in the gut, and the production of butyrate, supports overall BDNF levels.

feel-good chemicals

As mentioned in the previous chapter, our gut microbiota also produce and manage other 'feel-good' chemicals, such as the neurotransmitters serotonin, dopamine and GABA. GABA is the body's most important inhibitory neurotransmitter: it lowers neuronal activity and helps us feel less anxious; heightened anxiety can result in increased inflammation. Glutamate, which is the precursor to GABA, functions as a neurotransmitter involved in learning and memory, both of which can be impaired in neurodegenerative diseases such as Alzheimer's. Our gut microbiota has a crucial role in the production of these neurotransmitters, which is yet another reason to support it and help it to thrive.

Moreover, studies examining the composition of the gut microbiota in patients with depression demonstrated a predominance of potentially pathogenic and less beneficial bacteria that correlated with lower levels of serotonin. This has incredibly exciting implications for the role of gut-derived serotonin and its potential impact on mental wellbeing. In addition, lower amounts of dopamine have been observed in patients with depression – and, as mentioned previously, declining amounts of dopamine have also been linked with the development of certain neurodegenerative conditions, including Parkinson's.

This may have revolutionary implications for how we view and potentially include it as part of treating mood disorders and neurological conditions in the future – if the production of certain neurotransmitters in the gut can be manipulated. Through positively supporting

gut feelings

Some people do not experience any gut or digestive symptoms and may not be aware that their feelings of depression and/or anxiety could be deriving from an unhappy gut. While those with gut-related conditions such as irritable bowel syndrome (IBS) often notice that these symptoms co-exist, rarely is a patient who has depression or anxiety asked about the state of their gut health. This may be a vital link often missed in treatment. Indeed, there is often a mirroring of symptoms in the gut and the brain. For instance, when we have an excess of stress hormones, such as cortisol, and feel heightened anxiety, it typically manifests itself in an 'anxious gut', with cramping, urgency, pain and diarrhoea. Conversely, when we have low production of mood-enhancing neurotransmitters such as serotonin it can create a rather sluggish 'depressed gut', with symptoms like slow digestion and constipation that tend to correlate with a melancholic frame of mind. It seems our gut has feelings too.

our gut microbiota we may also be encouraging the production of more feel-good chemicals and an overall state of wellbeing. Happiness, it seems, is not just a state of mind but one of gut microbial temperament too.

age is but a number

The bond we have with our gut microbiome is one that is lifelong, deep and meaningful; it begins the moment we are born and continues until the end of our time on this earth. Just as we might notice changes in our appearance as we get older, changes in the make-up of the gut microbiome and the overall functioning of the gut are a natural part of the ageing process. And just as our obvious physical abilities, such as movement and muscle strength, wane as we get older, so too do our digestive powers.

When you think about the many psychological and physiological stressors that our gut microbes are presented with on a daily basis – the foods we do or don't eat, the medications we take and the general rigmarole of life – you can understand the immense hard work that our gut microbes have to put in to keep things on top form over the course of our lifetime.

As we age, the number of different species of bacteria residing in the gut naturally decreases. This seems to be particularly true of some of the butyrate-producing bacterial groups and, as I'm sure you'll have gathered by now, butyrate is super-important for both the gut and brain. Therefore, taking care of our gut microbiome throughout our life can serve us well. That means treating our trillions of life-long microbial companions with the love and respect they deserve, particularly in terms of the foods that support them; a topic we'll explore in the Chapter 6.

Unfortunately, we don't really help ourselves when it comes to preserving the variety and the 'youthful glow' of our gut microbiome as we age. Factors such as a diet that is lacking in dietary fibre and phytochemicals, certain medications, a lack of vitamin D and a life with too many worries can lower overall diversity of the gut microbiota. This lack of diversity

can also lead to a weakening of the gut barrier function and a compromised ability to manage inflammation. However, by supporting our gut microbiome over the years we can go some way towards mitigating the loss of species. So it's important to consider caring for our gut and our gut microbiome as part of a strategy for staying young in body and mind.

It's often said that you are only as old as you feel. When it comes to our gut microbiome, the sentiment is the same. If we can aim for an enriched existence for our gut microbes, we may also be able to maintain some of this youthful spark for our brain too.

keep calm and carry on

Throughout this chapter we have looked at the myriad ways that our gut and our gut microbiota help us to manage inflammation, and the role that this has to play in both mood and mindset. While the nutrients that we do, or don't, feed our gut microbiota can affect its ability to maintain a calmer situation in the body and brain, inflammation can equally result from a mind that is fraught with worries and stress.

Therefore maintaining a composed mindset is equally as important in order to support a tranquil state in the gut, and the rest of the body. That's why stress management, emotional support and learning to lean on others is so important. The next chapter will focus on reducing stress, another crucial factor in helping our trillions of microbes keep calm and carry on with their diligent work.

the stressed gut

ARE YOU BUSY, busy, busy? These days it has almost become a badge of honour to be seen to be as busy as possible. We might think that running at life a million miles an hour is the only way to achieve everything we need to – or think we need to – but, as Mahatma Gandhi said, 'There is more to life than increasing its speed.' When we continue in the rat race of life, trying to do too much day after day, there can be long-term and significant negative consequences for the health of our gut and our brain. Busy doesn't equal being happier and it can ultimately lead to a totally stressed-out state.

Chronic stress underpins countless modern diseases. It is particularly prevalent in those suffering from gut-related conditions such as IBS, so let's look at the effect that stress has on our gut microbiota and how trying to cope with our myriad pressures can profoundly alter their behaviour.

the stressful downward spiral

The gut and the brain communicate in various ways, as we discovered in Chapter 2. One of these – the HPA (hypothalamus-pituitary-adrenal) axis – relies on the endocrine system, the network of glands that release hormones into the bloodstream, and is pivotal to the stress response.

Chronic stress underpins countless modern diseases and is potentially one of the main causative factors.

As part of this response, the hypothalamus, the area of the brain that links the nervous and endocrine systems, reacts to 'foreign' substances and microbes circulating in the blood, as well as pro-inflammatory signals from the immune system. In response to this heightened inflammation, the hypothalamus sets off a cascade of alarm bells to the pituitary and adrenal glands, activating hormones such as noradrenaline and cortisol that elicit the stress, or fight or flight, response. We touched upon this earlier but it's worth repeating: this response is a natural reaction to stress and potential danger. It results in heightened alertness and an increased heart rate and blood flow to the arms and legs, making us better able to fight or flee. It is essentially our survival mechanism.

But here's the problem: the stress response essentially prioritises escaping or fighting the perceived threat over other systems in the body, including the functioning of the gut and the immune system. The reason for this is that digestion and immunity are of secondary concern when the body perceives there to be an imminent threat, because once the danger has passed our gut and immune system can, in

theory, resume normal duties. However, when we experience ongoing stress, the hormonal response is never switched off by the opposing so-called rest and digest mode that counterbalances it (see box on page 47). The constant stream of stress hormones that this causes, and the resulting chronic low-grade inflammation, can have a direct negative impact on the composition of gut microbiota.

Elevated cortisol may also increase the permeability of the gut barrier by triggering the release of pro-inflammatory cytokines and lipopolysaccharides (LPS) that can directly damage the gut lining, leading to a 'leaky gut'. This has the potential to escalate inflammation in the gut as well as overall low-grade chronic inflammation in the body, including the brain. As the gut becomes increasingly overwhelmed, more stress hormones and inflammatory signals are released, compromising both microbiota and barrier functioning of the gut. This perpetuates a downward spiral that puts a serious strain on the HPA axis.

To make matters worse, the chronic release of cortisol and noradrenaline can change intestinal secretions in the gut as a result of this low-grade chronic inflammation. This can alter gut acidity levels, making it a less hospitable environment for beneficial bacteria to live and thrive, but a nice spot for potential pathogens to set up home. This can also contribute to a state of dysbiosis in the gut microbiota which feeds back into this loop.

Furthermore, the alteration of these acids and secretions may impair the breakdown and absorption of food, resulting in digestive symptoms such as bloating, reflux and gas. Contrary to popular belief, it is very common for those who are under chronic stress and suffering from reflux-type symptoms to produce *inadequate* levels of stomach acid, rather than too much. If that rings a bell and you have spent years on various antacids, with little or no relief, maybe you need to think about reducing your stress levels, rather than your stomach acid.

It is evident that the brain has a significant effect on our stress response and how it impacts on our gut, but it works both ways. In fact, our gut microbiome can dictate how we respond to stressors.

a deeper sense of calm

The physical effects of stress can include nausea, diarrhoea and a generally unsettled gut. We may believe that such symptoms stem from the brain and psychological stressors but studies indicate that our gut microbiota can also help to control our body and brain's response to stress. Moreover, a gut microbiome that is lacking in beneficial bacteria may lead to a propensity for heightened stress reactions. One revealing study, published in *The Journal of Physiology,* demonstrated that germ-free mice (meaning they lack a microbiome) essentially overreacted and were hypersensitive to stress. They produced more cortisol, meaning that their HPA axis reaction was exaggerated, which resulted in a cascade of stress responses. What's even more fascinating is that when these same mice were fed a certain type of probiotic formula they appeared to become much calmer.

Another study observed that mice undergoing chronic stressors over a period of weeks showed a decrease in *lactobacilli* bacteria that correlated with an increase in depressive behaviour patterns; when probiotics were given the

behaviour patterns reversed. Of course, much research is still needed, and we are talking about mice; nevertheless, the implication that the composition of gut microbiota may have a role in regulating stress responses is pretty compelling.

Stress may have yet another connection to our microbiome. It has long been known that noradrenaline is a major chemical player in our fight or flight response, but what has recently become evident from several studies is that this same chemical can also be released in the gut and is in direct communication with gut microbiota. As you can imagine, a stress mediator chemical isn't likely to have a soothing effect on our gut microbes. In fact, it may stimulate the growth of pathogenic bacteria that have been linked to stomach ulcers and other gut infections. Moreover, not only does the release of noradrenaline increase the numbers of these potential pathogens but it also makes them more aggressive, so that they can maintain and increase their hold in the gut. In this case, it's survival of the most stressed-out bugs!

curb your adrenal spend

The adrenals are comparatively small glands that sit above our kidneys. Forming part of the trio in the HPA axis, these glands are the ones that produce hormones during periods of stress. As we saw in the previous chapter, it isn't just external psychological factors that lead us to a more stressed state, internal physiological stressors, such as gut inflammation or infections, elicit the same response from the HPA axis. The unfortunate irony here is that the more stressed we are

rest and digest

One of the most basic things that we can do to help manage stress is to consider meal times as dedicated and special moments in our day, rather than the rushed affairs that we often seem to make them. Placing a lot more importance on meal times as mini pockets of recovery allows us to properly 'rest and digest', rather than furiously gobbling down food, barely chewing it, while we pay more attention to the multiple electronic devices we have on the go. Destressing by using meal times as opportunities to get some time out from your day isn't adding in anything extra for you to think about. In fact, that's the whole point – that we should focus solely on our meal – no devices, no distractions.

The other stress we can put on the gut is getting into the habit of incessant grazing and snacking. Yes, a snack here and there is all well and good if we need it, but what I'm talking about is non-stop noshing. Rarely are we genuinely hungry when we are repeatedly reaching for snacks, and often this type of behaviour is more to do with reward-seeking or boredom. When we engage in this pattern of relentless feeding we are essentially asking the gut microbiome to work overtime. It is important to give your gut a bit of a rest between meals – ideally around 4–5 hours. Moreover, because we have some microbes that help us to absorb our food and others that come in for the 'clean-up' operation, they need some breathing space, just as we do, and I mean that quite literally.

If you think about it, periods of fasting are natural to all animals, including humans. It is only in recent decades that we have had constant access to foods such as sweet treats and salty snacks. In earlier times there was always a clear break between meals and, going back even further, our ancestors may simply not have had any food available when they wanted it. Studies have shown that fasting periods can have a range of health benefits, including improving the balance of microbes in the gut, reducing the risk of type-2 diabetes and a reduction in belly fat.

psychologically, the less well placed we are to deal with physiological stressors. Stress is part of life, and a healthy part at that, but not when it is relentless and pronounced.

Knowingly and persistently hammering your adrenals, which manage these stress hormones, is something that we can take ownership of and address if we want to better support the HPA axis and its relationship with our gut. When stress hormones such as cortisol are chronically activated, there is also an effect on insulin, the hormone that manages blood sugar (glucose) levels by shuttling glucose into our cells. On the face of it, cortisol and insulin might appear to be in total opposition and that is certainly the case when we are in an acute stressful situation: we release cortisol, blood sugar levels increase and glucose is mobilised ready to help us fight or run. Once the threat is over, blood sugar levels drop back down. However, when stress is chronic, glucose levels remain high and, without physical exertion to burn off this glucose, the release of insulin is triggered. When cortisol is chronically elevated it can lead to increased insulin and ultimately insulin resistance, where the body essentially stops responding to the signals of insulin. This cortisol–insulin imbalance can create a propensity to gain weight around the middle, often referred to as 'stress belly'.

Moreover, if we remain on the same stress loop, constantly stimulating the adrenals to produce these hormones, it can lead into a dysfunctional HPA axis and an imbalance in cortisol production. This is often referred to as adrenal fatigue. It will almost always begin with an overactivation of stress hormones, which can be self-perpetuating – adrenaline junkie sound familiar? However, after some time your adrenals will not be able to keep up with the constant demand for these stress hormones, resulting in 'adrenal fatigue'. And you will feel pretty damn tired, that's for sure. You are also likely to experience symptoms such as loss of libido, poor sleep, food cravings and, to top it all, the 'stress belly' effect mentioned above.

It's vital then to begin addressing the factors that are causing you stress *before* you reach the stage where you have utterly exhausted your adrenals. Some of these factors will be more obvious and indeed easier to tackle than others: for example, changing career might not be easy but things like not getting enough or decent quality sleep, skipping meals and overdoing it on the caffeine and booze will all put pressure on the adrenals. By starting with what might seem like one minor change you can take many positive steps towards a significant reduction in stress overall.

Choosing the types of food that encourage more 'stress-busting' beneficial bugs to flourish

is an integral part of this. I will outline the gut-microbiome-nourishing foods we should all be eating in Chapter 6, but it's also helpful to be aware of some specific foods that can help us towards a less frazzled state, and the ones that might well be fuelling our stress. While I am not suggesting that simply eating some foods and avoiding others is a cure-all for stress, it can certainly be useful in helping us towards a more calm existence

What can we do then, in terms of our diet, to ease the stress?

stress less menu

At the heart of a 'stress less' menu from a gut perspective should be a focus on supporting and nourishing our gut microbiota with its favourite flavours. This includes myriad sources of dietary fibre, with diversity in the colour and types of vegetables, fruit, wholegrains, nuts and seeds eaten. Complementing this are fermented foods that are rich in beneficial microbes such as live yogurts, cheese, sauerkraut and kimchi. Foods that are high in omega-3 essential fatty acids also have a fundamental role in how we manage stress, both by supporting brain function and mood and in their general anti-inflammatory effect. The best sources of these foods are outlined in detail in Chapter 6. However, I have outlined below some particular nutrients that could help us move towards a less stressed state.

Foods high in vitamin C Vitamin C is a key component in the production of adrenal hormones, and is used up rapidly when we are pumping them out incessantly. The other crucial role that vitamin C plays is supporting the production of collagen, which helps to maintain healthy connective tissue, including that of the gut barrier. Foods that are high in vitamin C include peppers, broccoli and other green vegetables, kiwi fruit and berries. Also, baobab powder, derived from the baobab fruit, (which we'll look at more in Chapter 6 and is also featured in a few of the recipes) is valuable in this respect. It's also a simple, stress-free addition to breakfasts and puddings.

Foods high in vitamin B5 Avocado is a rich source of vitamin C and it also boasts high levels of B vitamins, in particular pantothenic acid, or vitamin B5, a favoured nutrient for the adrenal glands. Sunflower seeds are another excellent source of B5 so sprinkle them through roasted vegetables and salads or on top of your morning oats. And if you are a fan of chicken liver this is a true winner in the B5 stakes; it also contains many other B vitamins, iron and vitamin A that can all benefit the gut and the adrenals. Just ensure you buy free-range livers and avoid them during pregnancy. If the idea of cooking chicken liver is intimidating, start with the spag bol recipe on page 169, which I've tinkered with to include liver and more fibre than the standard version.

Foods high in magnesium Magnesium is top of the league when it comes to calming the nerves – and it is a mineral that our body tends to use up in large quantities during stressful periods. You'll find it in nuts and seeds, whole grains, avocados and leafy greens.

Mean greens To complete your calming menu, try to eat more leafy greens such as spinach, rainbow chard, kale, rocket and cavolo nero. These provide a veritable feast of nutrients, such as B vitamins, magnesium, fibre and antioxidants, that all help to reduce overall stress on the gut, brain and adrenals.

buzz foods

On the flip side there are foods that can leave us highly strung when we overindulge in them. As outlined earlier, in the normal stress reaction, the body releases the hormone cortisol in response to sudden stress, counteracting insulin (the hormone that regulates blood-sugar levels) and immediately raising our blood sugar. Excessive amounts of sugar can upset the balance of the relationship between insulin and cortisol. Moreover, long-term stress can cause chronically elevated levels of cortisol, so the body stops responding to insulin signals and this can develop into insulin resistance. This essentially means that our cells become resistant to insulin's instructions to store sugar for energy use and instead it is converted into fat that typically sits around the belly area.

Now that's not to say that the odd dessert here and there can't be part of a balanced diet, and is actually part of the joy of eating, but furiously gobbling up chocolate, cookies and cakes in response to stress is something else. Furthermore, high cortisol combined with high insulin levels will create more of a need for high-fat and high-sugar foods, which is part of the reason for so-called 'stress eating'. Therefore, it isn't helpful simply to say 'eat less sugar', because unless we manage stress we will naturally gravitate towards sugary foods. If this sounds familiar, try to pinpoint when and why you have compelling urges towards this pattern and work on those triggers, (using professional support where you need it) rather than denying yourself sugar altogether. We can certainly have our cake and eat it without feeling like the cake has got the better of us.

The other habit many of us get into when stressed is loading up on coffee or caffeinated tea to get us through the day. Coffee, when it is the proper fresh stuff, and good quality tea, do have some bona fide benefits for the gut, brain health and in managing stress because they contain polyphenols and antioxidants that help to support the microbiome, as well as mitigating damage and stress to cells. However, we can definitely have too much of a good thing. The reason why we feel instantly energised from caffeine is that it increases stress hormones like cortisol and adrenaline. Great when we need a spurt of energy and can then allow our bodies to go back to a more rested state. Not so great when we are in a constant adrenaline-fuelled state that keeps us permanently in fight or flight mode. Having a couple of cups per day, if you are not jittery from way too much stress, can be part of a healthy approach to caffeine. Try to have caffeine after breakfast when you have food in your belly to avoid spiking stress hormones further. And avoid having caffeine late in the day as it can affect sleep, and a lack of decent quality zzzs can be just as much of a hit to the adrenals as it is to the gut and brain. It's best to enjoy your daily cuppa as the sun rises and not in the twilight hours.

Evenings are often the time when we fancy a tipple or two. Now I'm not shy about enjoying a glass of wine and there are legit benefits to having some beneficial polyphenols in vino form … OK so you can get way more antioxidants from other foods but suffice to say enjoying a glass of wine here and there in moderation is one of the joys of life. And, of course, a glass of your preferred drink can take the edge off stress and alleviate pressure. It becomes an issue when it is the excessive, chronic and dependent type of drinking that impacts the entire body … and I don't need to tell you about the squiffy effects it has on the brain.

When it comes to booze, we need to be mindful of the type of alcohol we consume and the circumstances in which we are drinking. Accompanying a delicious meal, catching up with friends, toasting and celebrating moments of life are how we can best use and appreciate booze. Scheduling dedicated 'dry' days is a good tactic too. I rather like the 3:3 rule that Rosamund Dean suggests in her book *Mindful Drinking:* having three days a week that you can enjoy alcohol but sticking to no more than three drinks on those days. I think that's pretty doable and means that we can enjoy the benefits without the brutal after-effects of one (or three) too many!

go your own way

Managing stress from a microbiota–gut–brain perspective requires us to better nourish and be kind to our mind *and* our gut microbiota. It isn't enough to practise meditation and deep breathing, for example, without thinking about the health of our gut and being mindful of the stress that negatively impacts our gut microbiota. Equally, focusing only on our gut health and hoping that our gut microbiota will calm our mind is just as myopic. We are all individuals and can choose to be busy with the things, people and situations that provide us with satisfaction, rather than staying on the demanding treadmill of stress. As Hans Selye, the scientist who conducted pioneering research into the effects of stress, said, 'It's not stress that kills us, it is our reaction to it.' Take life at a slower pace, be less busy and make the race the one that you really want to win, and not one you unintentionally find yourself competing in.

sweet dreams

WE'VE ALL BEEN there after a bad night's sleep – exhausted, confused, weak, achy, foggy and generally off-kilter. We might have been tossing, turning and ruminating over worries that, in the middle of the night, feel insurmountable. Or perhaps it was due to too many cups of coffee, leaving us wide awake when we should be happily snoozing away. Poor, fragmented or even a total lack of sleep are common complaints, and while the odd sleepless night is one thing, a chronic pattern of under-sleeping can result in much more serious side effects than just feeling a bit more lethargic, unfocused and irritable the following day.

Sometimes it is easy to pinpoint what caused a restless night but there can be underlying health factors that affect the general quality and quantity of our sleep.

One of these is the health of our gut, more specifically the gut microbiota. Indeed, compelling scientific research is emerging which suggests that there is a crucial connection between the health of the gut microbiome and sleep, so in this chapter we will be 'getting into bed' with our gut bugs and looking at their ability to influence pillow time.

our body clock

On average, most adults need around seven to eight hours of good-quality sleep every night in order to be well refreshed and fully functioning the next day. Some people are fine with a bit less and some need a bit more. You'll know if you are falling short on sleep if you generally feel exhausted throughout the day and an afternoon nap becomes a prerequisite. The fact is that, due to our busy lives, we commonly override our natural instinct to go to sleep when we are tired. Instead, with the backdrop of blue lights from myriad devices, we tend to go against our natural sleeping patterns and favour scrolling and liking over pillow time, well into the twilight hours. We essentially fight our biochemical internal clock, which operates over a 24-hour period, known as a circadian rhythm, and regulates our sleep–wake cycle.

It works like this. In the morning the sleep hormone melatonin lowers, we wake up, our gut readies itself to eliminate toxins, cortisol produced by our adrenal glands spurs us to start the day, ready for action, and our pancreas produces insulin in anticipation of the breakfast we are about to eat. The earlier part of the day is also when our brain is at peak performance, while the afternoon is the time when our muscle tone reaches its full potential. As the day comes to an end, cortisol falls and melatonin rises to lull us to sleep. Healthy sleep works in phases of deep sleep interspersed with REM (rapid eye movement) sleep; these phases occur three to five times per night, in approximately 90-minute cycles.

You might naturally assume that while we sleep our internal clock is letting our body gently tick over. In fact, the brain does a lot while we are snoozing away, blissfully unaware. It produces hormones such as melatonin and human growth hormone, as well as doing what could be best described as a general 'clean-up' operation to eliminate toxins. Human growth hormone also stimulates the renewal and replacement of damaged cells throughout the body, including those of the gut barrier. This general clean-up is mirrored by our gut microbes, in that the gut microbiota uses the time we are asleep to do its own housekeeping. Sleep is therefore vital for our entire body to repair, regenerate and restore.

Working against our natural circadian rhythm means we create more of a discord in its rhythms. Repeatedly disrupting our internal clock potentially sets up our entire system for multiple failures. The results of being 'off' our biological beat, and the resulting build-up of sleep deprivation, are typically more frequent bouts of sickness, poor decision-making, and gut-related symptoms such as queasiness and general malaise. These might seem like trivial health niggles but in the longer term they can contribute to much more serious health conditions, including heart disease, diabetes and obesity.

Part of this discord of rhythms also links with the disordered timing of our food intake, as we can literally have food at our fingertips 24/7. Eating at random times can put our natural biological clock out of order and that can impact on metabolism and digestive processes, regardless of what we are actually eating. It seems that many of us have lost touch with our body's natural rhythms, including those of our gut microbiome. When you consider that pretty much every living thing follows natural rhythmic cycles, it is rather arrogant to think that we can go so far off the beat and not feel out of sync.

bedtime bugs

While there are sometimes obvious factors that can disrupt our sleep, such as late-night coffee consumption or a night on the tiles, there is a considerable amount of research to suggest that the health of our gut microbiome may also have a significant impact on the sleep–wake cycle. It seems as though microbial life has its own daily rhythms that work harmoniously with circadian rhythms and that one has the capacity to alter and disturb the other.

Many of us have lost touch with our body's natural rhythms, including those of our gut microbiome.

The daily rhythms of the gut microbiome are largely shaped by the timing and the type of foods we eat. We also know that the composition of our microbiome changes in response to feeding and fasting (for example, overnight), as we have some microbes that help us to absorb and digest our food and others that prefer a fasted state so that they can get on with the task of cleaning up: this is why diversity in the microbiome is so crucial for our gut. It also works the other way around in that disruptions to circadian rhythms, such as jet lag, can disrupt the rhythm and health of our microbiome. You may have noticed that it can take your gut a while to adjust to a new time zone; the common symptoms in reaction to this being indigestion and constipation. Either way, a gut microbiota that is out of balance can confuse communication between the gut and the brain, which can have a direct impact on sleep.

Indeed, you might say that the microbiota–gut–brain connection has a rhythm of its own, and our gut microbiota has both a direct and indirect impact on sleep. One key aspect to bear in mind is the influence that our gut microbiota has on mood and emotional wellbeing. As we saw in Chapter 3, anxiety and depression can create or increase disrupted and disordered sleep patterns.

Another important connection, and a very common factor in impaired sleep, is stress. The relationship between stress and the gut is closely intertwined: a stressed gut microbiome can lead to a stressed mind and vice versa. The hormone cortisol is released by the adrenal glands in the morning, as part of the natural sleep–wake cycle, but is also released in response to stress, as discussed in the previous chapter. When stress becomes chronic, excess cortisol, combined with the worries themselves, will very likely hinder us from sleeping well since cortisol keeps us alert. If someone is in a pattern where the adrenals are pumping out too much cortisol, they may tend to wake up in the early hours of the morning, around 2–4am, since this is when cortisol naturally starts to rise. Furthermore, high cortisol levels can impair diversity in the gut microbiota and compromise the gut barrier. Managing your stress is therefore an important part of getting your sleep sorted.

The health of our gut can also affect our sleep due to increased inflammation. When the gut microbiota is compromised this can impair the way that our body deals with inflammation – and an inflamed system is not going to allow us to rest well. Further to this, lack of sleep, especially in the most restorative phase of deep sleep, doesn't allow our gut microbiota sufficient time to do what they need to do when we are sleeping, including secreting substances that help to manage inflammation. This can be detrimental not just to the gut but to the entire body, including the brain.

Having a good night's sleep also crucially relies on the production of our natural sedative hormones and neurotransmitters, which are not only produced in our brain but also by the trillions of microbes in our gut. GABA (gamma-amino butyric acid) is the body's most important inhibitory neurotransmitter, which means it reduces the activity of neurons in the brain and the central nervous system, and has a calming effect that supports healthy sleep. Basically, GABA helps to lull both the gut and the brain to a more restful night. Lower amounts of GABA have been observed in those who suffer from insomnia and fragmented sleep.

The other hormone that is vital for the sleep–wake cycle is melatonin, aka 'the hormone of darkness' since it is higher in the evening. When the sun goes down the pineal gland in the brain begins to produce melatonin, which makes us feel sleepy. Interestingly melatonin is not only produced in the brain but also in the gut to create a more localised calming effect.

You can now begin to appreciate that our gut may have a significant role in how well we sleep, and have a better understanding of the intricate ways in which our gut microbiota move to a similar beat to that of our circadian rhythm. It may be that developing better sleeping habits relies, in part, on being more in tune with our gut bugs.

perfect timing

It is obvious that the erratic and frenetic way in which we live our lives can affect the quality and quantity of our sleep. Factors such as changes in timing of meals, which could include skipping meals or eating late at night, too much or too little physical exercise, putting in countless hours of overtime and frequent travelling can all take us away from a pattern that flows with our natural rhythm. Constantly changing and shifting routines can create disharmony with circadian rhythms and leave our system confused. Ultimately, the discord between the innate timings of our circadian rhythms and how we approach life can result in a lack of good quality sleep, and the associated negative knock-on effects.

It makes sense that we should want to optimise activities such as eating, sleeping and moving, in order to maximise our performance, and much of that does depend on adhering to our natural rhythms. It doesn't really take much for us to comprehend that just as our mind is tired by the end of the day, so too is our gut and its trillions of microbial residents. Motility, the movement of food and waste material through the gut, slows down into the night, which is part of the reason we can usually sleep for seven or eight hours without needing to go poop, but is also why we might experience symptoms such as bloating and indigestion as a result of eating too late. Going to bed when your last meal hasn't been properly digested is not going to make for a good night's sleep. Saliva production reduces markedly into the evening and when we are asleep: if you are suffering heartburn at night and are eating late, this could be one factor to bear in mind, because saliva helps to neutralise acid that causes reflux. Also, eating late into the evening makes our gut work 'overtime' and that can have negative consequences on the gut microbiota and in turn on circadian rhythms and the sleep–wake cycle.

There is a lot to be said about timing. Try to make breakfast or lunch your biggest meal, as the earlier part of the day is when insulin sensitivity is higher, which helps to better manage your blood-sugar levels throughout the day. Dinner is when we tend to eat with family and friends (hopefully!) and spending time together is an important part of overall health and wellbeing. The earlier you can do this the better. Allow at least two to three hours after your last bite, or drink of anything other than water, in the evening before you go to bed. Whatever you consume on waking, even if it's just a cup of coffee, will start your 'gut clock' again.

The daily rhythms of the gut microbiome are largely shaped by the timing and the type of foods we eat.

Ideally we want to aim for a 12 to 15-hour period of not eating or drinking anything other than water: this will help to keep our circadian rhythms in sync. For most of us this is perfectly doable, for example between 8pm and 8am. This has been referred to as Time Restricted Eating, or TRE. It's not a new idea: overnight fasting gives our digestion and gut a rest so that in the morning we are ready for breakfast – 'breaking the fast'.

In general, try to keep to a regular schedule of eating so that your gut knows when to expect food. This helps to maintain rhythm with your bowel movements, as well as your circadian rhythms and gut microbiome. TRE also allows our gut microbes to perform the crucial processes of cleaning up and clearing out that can have such positive effects on the gut and those systems linked to the gut, such as the immune system and the brain. I would go further and suggest sticking to three meals a day that you try to eat at around the same times. The gut and the gut microbiota like a regular routine and random eating could potentially be a significant factor in a gut that is behaving erratically. It's just common sense really. The more you eat in an erratic way, the more you are cultivating a gut microbiota that is out of sync, and that can create symptoms such as erratic sleep.

sleep stealers

While keeping to daily rhythms and routines can go a long way towards improving our sleep, we also need to address some of the specific factors that might be causing us to count sheep way into the early hours.

worries and woes

We have already touched on the physical effects of stress on the gut microbiome and the sleep–wake cycle. Stress can often present itself as insomnia, either the inability to get to sleep or waking in the night and struggling to get back to sleep. If you feel that this has become a feature for you then now is the time to address the ongoing stressors in your life. However, it can be hard to pinpoint psychological stressors. If we know what is keeping us up at night then worrying incessantly isn't going to solve the problem, but tangibly trying to do something about it can. Obviously, some stressors can be harder than others to positively shift, but just asking for help and having a plan can at least start the process for a lot of us. That alone can lift some of the worrisome burden. Meditation and mindfulness practices can also be a good starting point (see page 83) and while they cannot always remove the stress they can certainly help us to deal with it better.

energy fixers

Another very common sleep saboteur is consuming lots of high-energy food and drinks, such as sugary snacks, junk food, fizzy drinks and coffee. It is relatively easy to get into a negative feedback loop with these kinds of foods and the associated cravings.

When we are not sleeping and are feeling tired it seems to make sense to have something that will provide an immediate 'fix'. However, a high intake of sugar, ultra-processed junk foods and caffeine can mask genuine fatigue, so we get less rest and end up more sleep deprived. Often we then compensate by eating more of these foods to get energy, further disrupting our sleep. Sleep deprivation also directly affects hunger and satiety hormones: a sleepless night can lead to a surge in ghrelin, the hormone that tells our brain that we are hungry, and/or a fall in leptin, which tells us that we are full. As a result we may be overeating due to these hormones being out of sync.

So what can you do?

- Restrict your intake of caffeine (from tea, coffee and 'energy drinks') to no later than midday, and stick to no more than two to three cups per day on average. If you are particularly sensitive to the effects of caffeine then reduce further.

- Try to eat three meals a day and avoid skipping meals as that may mean that you end up reaching for a sugary snack. Include plenty of complex carbohydrates in these meals, such as whole grains, oats, quinoa, buckwheat, spelt, wild rice or sourdough, along with some kind of protein, as that will help to keep you better satiated.

- If you tend to need a snack in the afternoon, plan it so that you don't go for whatever is hanging around the office or in the kids' treats drawer. Something like half an avocado sprinkled with seeds or an oatcake with some cheese could be good options.

- Consider including foods that can help to promote better sleep, such as natural sources of GABA (the 'calming' neurotransmitter) – green, black and oolong tea, milk kefir, 'live' yogurt and tempeh – and foods that can boost our own production, such as lentils, walnuts, almonds, fish, berries, spinach, broccoli, potatoes and cocoa.

- And, of course, ensure that your meals include a diversity of fibre and fermented foods to support the health of your gut microbiota.

booze

You don't really need me to tell you about the other major sleep disruptor – alcohol. None of us sleep better when we've had a few too many. This is because alcohol is a diuretic so it makes us want to pee more and that can cause us to wake in the night. It also directly disrupts the hormones that govern the sleep–wake cycle by producing a chemical called adenosine: this makes us feel sleepy, so we go to sleep, but then wake before being fully rested. We end up in less of the restful, and more time in the REM, stage of sleep and will feel tired no matter how long we stay in bed.

While a glass of wine with dinner for those who enjoy it is generally fine, too much isn't a good thing, and using wine or beer to help us get to sleep is not a good idea. We might assume that alcohol is a relaxant but it can act as a stimulant too. For nights off, try a sparkling water with lemon juice in a wine glass – for the psychological effect – or even something like water kefir (see page 204), which is like champagne for the gut!

being too sedentary

Food and drink aside, a lack of physical exercise can affect the way we sleep. If we are sitting down all day we may simply not be physically tired. Being overly sedentary reduces our body's production of growth hormones that promote sleep (which are increased in response to exercise). You don't need to be working out to the point of exhaustion but regular daily movement can help to support better and deeper sleep. Walking is a great form of physical activity because it gets us outside and in natural light which leads nicely onto the next sleep stealer…

artificial light

The reality is that many of us are spending more time in artificial light, which is not conducive to helping us to sleep better. When we are awake we might spend most of the day in offices with very little exposure to natural light. It's no wonder the brain loses its concept of time, and that can mess up our sleep patterns. We also know that vitamin D, which we predominantly get from sunlight exposure, is important for many reasons relating to the health of our body, brain and gut. Try to get some natural light as soon as you wake up but, if that's not possible, at least at some point during the day. Resist the temptation to work through lunch at your

desk, for example, and instead get some fresh air outside to help reset your mind, gut and circadian rhythms.

Quiet time to yourself is vital, and you can make a start by setting some boundaries to the onslaught of the virtual world so that you can rest and reflect.

digital devices

Probably the most significant sleep stealer in our modern lifestyles is that of digital screens and the virtual world. This follows no rhythm or timetable whatsoever: it is constantly active and we can engage with it any time we choose. The more we keep ourselves awake looking at devices the less we are promoting sleep. Blue-light exposure late into the evening is particularly disruptive, although nowadays it is very straightforward to download apps that can help to reduce this on your phone, tablet and laptop, and many of them have it built in as a feature. However, dimmers aside, there is a need to put a curfew on this stuff and to engage only when and where it is appropriate, for the sake of our sleep and our sanity. Frankly, the bedroom should be a place that is used for only two things and neither of them is shopping on the internet or checking social media. Avoid using mobiles as alarm clocks; instead, get an old-fashioned clock and switch your phone off and put it in another room when you go to bed. The ritual of doing that will also signal that you need to recharge properly too, and take the time to let your mind settle before bed. Quiet time

rock-a-bye baby

If we are not sleeping enough then there is one very obvious way to right this – get more sleep! For some of us it might not be so straightforward, but for many there are factors that we can change to help with this. It also isn't the case of banking sleep on the weekend and then powering through the week, burning the candle at both ends and surviving on much less sleep. It really requires us to prioritise our pillow time more consistently. We cannot stimulate our brain, gut and overall system right up until we decide to go to sleep and then expect to be happily snoozing away moments later. Creating a pre-bedtime routine is a necessary part of helping to get our mind and body ready for sleep.

Take the hour before you go to bed to remove stress – and that includes the anxiety around getting to sleep. That might mean writing down concerns and 'brain dumping' from the day so that you alleviate this stress rather than it swirling around in your mind. Instead create a soothing cocoon, for example by taking a warm bath, reading a book or doing some meditation or deep breathing exercises.

Removing all electrical appliances from the bedroom is certainly a must and, with that, turning off your phone an hour before bedtime to allow your mind and body to wind down properly. There are very few emails, texts or WhatsApp messages that cannot wait until the morning. Creating the right ambience in the bedroom means curtains or blinds that effectively shut out street lights and a temperature that is not too warm, as that can also affect sleep. If you need ear plugs (a snoring partner or noisy neighbours) and/or an eye mask to help you really detach from the buzzing of the outside world then use them. Then just let the magic happen and await a blissful night ahead.

to yourself is vital, and you can make a start by setting some boundaries to the onslaught of the virtual world so that you can rest and reflect.

night night…

As we put this topic to bed, take a moment to reflect on how the power of our gut and the trillions of microbes that we go to sleep with on a nightly basis can lend us a more restful slumber. The effect of our gut microbiota on pillow time is one that is much more profound and remarkable than we might have considered. In working with the rhythm of our gut microbiome, and nourishing it well, we can skip to a similar beat as our circadian rhythms and waltz with our microbes to a better night's sleep. Sweet dreams…

eat well

WHEN WE HAPPILY tuck into a meal how many of us think beyond the foods that we like to enjoy and that suit our palette? We eat what *we* want, right? Well, we could dine solely for our own delight, but it's not very considerate to the trillions of microbes that dine with us at each meal. If we want to aim for a happier gut, and a happier mind, when deciding on the foods that grace our plate we also need to take into consideration those that tickle the taste buds of our gut microbiota.

There are no two ways about it, food, and the experience of eating, is intrinsic to the meaning of life, including the buoyant existence of our gut microbiota. In a matter of decades we have swapped a culture around food that was based on natural, seasonal, largely local produce, and eating together, for one that is in many ways entirely 'unnatural', with excessive amounts of calories and ultra-processed foods, where convenience is the main priority. But, as we will see, convenience comes at a cost for our inner microbial life.

Yes, the typical Western diet can appear appetising and attractive, but it can often be decidedly lacking in fibre and loaded with chemicals to make the food look good and taste more palatable. These fibre-devoid foods are anything but enticing for our gut microbes. Their preferred menu would look strikingly different – it would be full of veg, fruits, nuts, seeds and wholegrains that are rich in dietary fibre and phytonutrients (those wonderful disease-fighting compounds found in plant-based foods). Fermented foods would also be on the daily specials board, to add extra microbes to the mix.

So, what constitutes a good diet for our gut microbiota? To answer that question, we can take a look back at the diet of our distant ancestors. Thankfully we are able to do that to some degree by looking at hunter-gatherer communities that still exist, like the Hadza tribe in East Africa, who adhere to a very traditional way of eating and whose gut health has been the focus of much research.

step back in time

The Hadza follow a lifestyle that is little changed from that of our hunter-gatherer ancestors some tens of thousands of years ago, and as a result they have an incredibly diverse gut microbiota. Their diet is very varied and abundant in plant foods that provide many different types of fibre and phytonutrients.

The Hadza depend entirely on what is naturally available when they forage and hunt. As the seasons change, so too do the plants in season, which provides them with a naturally diverse range of dietary fibre over the course of the year. The amount of meat that they consume also varies, as the dry season makes for more successful hunting. This means that, overall, their diet contains very modest amounts of

healthy fats, fish and meat. They also eat wild honey, but, as with meat, this is something they need to work hard to obtain. This is very different from our 'convenient' Western diet, which tends to feature the same vegetables and fruit week in week out, flown from the other side of the world, which means that they can be lower in some nutrients. Our diet is also characterised by our seemingly insatiable – and unsustainable – *over*consumption of food.

Obviously not everyone in the western world is living on a junk food diet, but the stark reality is that a large proportion of us are not eating enough plant-based foods or a varied enough selection. This means that we are depriving ourselves of the dietary fibre and phytochemicals that we, and our gut microbes, need. The most important lesson from the research on the Hadza is that increasing our intake of plant-based foods and eating less – but better quality – meat will support and potentially transform the health of our gut microbiome.

Scientists who analysed the composition of the gut microbiome of the Hadza, and compared them with typical Western ones, found that not only do they have a far greater number of beneficial bacteria, but they also have a much wider biodiversity than our urban version. It seems that we have lost up to a third of our gut microbial diversity. That's a hell of a lot and a rather worrying observation when you consider just how much we depend on our gut microbes.

Further to this the Hadza are free from the chronic health conditions and mood disorders, such as depression and anxiety, that are massively on the rise in the Western world. Of course, this isn't down to diet alone. When it comes to exercise, the Hadza are not running bleary-eyed on a treadmill or sitting on a stationary bike, and neither are they sedentary for long periods. Walking for several hours a day is natural to them, as most of their time is spent sourcing food. Social interaction and collaboration are crucial in foraging, hunting and cooking, and their strong sense of community is fundamental to their emotional wellbeing.

While we can't replicate the way of life in such tribes, and I'm not suggesting you forage for your supper, there are lessons we can learn from them if we want to emulate their rich and dynamic gut microbiome.

a meal fit for gut microbes

That age-old saying 'you are what you eat' isn't really that accurate. Well, not at least as far as our gut microbiota are concerned. We have to consider the meals we are providing for our gut microbes, as well as our own personal taste, if we want a satisfied and satiated gut microbiota. Feeding our gut microbes and satisfying their appetite is a key part of helping to cultivate a gut and mind that is full of *joie de vivre*. So what foods should we be focusing on?

you are what your microbes eat

One of the main ingredients in the recipe for a healthy gut microbiota is dietary fibre. While our digestive system doesn't have the capability to digest fibre, it provides a veritable feast for our gut microbiota, enabling it to produce beneficial substances such as SCFAs, which have a significant role in the health of our gut

and brain. Dietary fibre is found in all plant-based carbohydrates, encompassing all types of vegetables, fruit, whole grains, nuts and seeds – and each plant food contains different types of fibre. Just as we have penchants for different flavours, so does our gut microbiota: different gut microbes can have preferences for the type of fibre they like to eat. The key thing to aim for is diversity in our intake, rather than focusing on quantity alone. Each plant food will contain various types of dietary fibre so, for example, oats provide beta-glucan, legumes like lentils, beans and peas have raffinose in abundance and cereal grains are loaded with lignin. In providing these different types of fibre for our gut microbes we help to create an overall more heterogeneous and healthier gut microbiota.

In general, dietary fibre consumption has markedly decreased in recent years, in part due to the increased intake of ultra-processed food (see page 68). This essentially starves the gut microbiome of its favoured sustenance. But we can change that.

Current guidelines suggest that adults should eat around 30 grams of dietary fibre per day. In real terms that could equate in total to something like one piece of fruit, six portions of vegetables, two servings of wholegrains and three portions of nuts and seeds. That may seem quite a task but if you think about adding a spoonful of nut butter to porridge oats, along with a serving of berries, sprinkling seeds over your salads and vegetables and aiming for a mix of three types of veggies at lunch and supper you have pretty much hit your quota. The other key point to remember is that the more we can mix up our repertoire of fibre, the more we are supporting a diversity of microbes in our gut, which means a healthier gut overall.

Practically that could mean putting a different fruit or veg into your weekly shop, rotating your regular morning oats with other grains such as spelt, rye, buckwheat, quinoa or millet, using a variety of frozen berries and having a few flavours of nut and seed butters that you can mix and match.

If you also want to reflect elements of the Hadza diet, and hopefully their gut microbiome, you could include some of their preferred types of food in your weekly shop. This could be tuber vegetables such as sweet potatoes, Jerusalem artichokes, cassava, yams and tiger nuts. You could also think about adding baobab powder to your breakfast: the fruit of the baobab tree is a traditional part of the Hadza diet and it contains a high amount of fibre and vitamin C. It has a slightly sour yet sweet zingy taste that some people liken to sherbet. I reckon it's ace blended with bananas (you'll find a simple yet versatile recipe for this on page 176).

A word of warning: for some people, particularly those suffering from conditions like irritable bowel syndrome (IBS), it is important to be mindful of the type of fibre as well as volume. Some people can react very badly to high amounts of fibre, so go easy with it if you are not used to it, and introduce new types gently. This is especially true for some of the more potent fibrous foods which we will come on to next.

prebiotics

Prebiotics are types of dietary fibre that have an enhanced feeding effect on beneficial gut microbes. Currently, there is evidence that three main prebiotics can have a positive effect on our gut microbiota: inulin, fructooliogosaccharide (FOS) and galactooligosaccharide (GOS). These can be found in thousands of foods including top hitters such as garlic, onions, leeks, Jerusalem artichokes, asparagus, almonds, cashews, pistachios, mushrooms and wholegrains including sourdough. Chicory root is a particularly rich source of inulin, although it's not the easiest ingredient to incorporate into the diet: try it in my Maca Mocha (page 193).

Another substance that acts like a prebiotic fibre but isn't referred to as such is *resistant starch*. This is found in foods such as cooked and cooled white potatoes, legumes like lentils and chickpeas, and under-ripe bananas.

what the ferment?

Fermentation and fermented foods have been given a trendy renaissance in recent years, but it's a process that has been an intrinsic part of a diverse range of cultures for centuries. Think Korean kimchi, Japanese miso, Russian kvass, sauerkraut, or 'kraut as it's more affectionately known by my Polish ancestors, and, closer to home, 'live' yogurt and cheese. Traditionally, fermented foods played a more significant role in our diet, as our ancestors used this method to preserve foods, but with the introduction of fridges and other such appliances we lost the need to practise this technique. Until, that is, it found its way back into popular culture, and culture really is the apropos word.

culture club

The main thing to bear in mind is that fermentation fundamentally relies on the presence of a thriving set of live microbes. It is mostly an anaerobic process, which means that it doesn't use oxygen. It is in fact the happy end product of a multitude of microbes that essentially 'pre-digest' food and liquids into their fermented forms.

This can either be based on a specific 'starter culture' of microbes to kick-start the process of fermentation or left more to microbial 'chance'. Culture-based fermented foods typically include most cheese, yogurt and milk/water kefirs – these rely on kefir-grain starters that look a bit alien-like. Kombucha, which is a fizzy fermented tea, also relies on a starter culture called a SCOBY, an acronym for symbiotic culture of bacteria and yeast. Kefir and kombucha might sound a tad disconcerting but once you try them you'll find them rather pleasing.

The other type of fermentation is the result of spontaneous microbes that already exist on the surface of plants and in the air; often called 'wild fermentation' or 'wild airborne fermentation', this is how most vegetables and grains, as in the case of sourdough, are fermented, although starter cultures can also be used to speed this process up and gain uniformity of taste and quality.

In order for these microbes to perform the task of fermenting they need to be given a source of 'food' as fuel. Depending on the type of food you wish to ferment, this will require different microbes that provide them with their favourite type of food. For instance, microbes

chicken soup for the soul?

The bone broth trend shows no sign of disappearing fast but it's not some new, hip food. My nan will be almost certainly be looking down on the trend with some bewilderment. She used bone broth, or 'stock' as she called it, as a base for many a dish, so it would have been incomprehensible that there was such a flurry of attention around something that was pretty standard for her to make on a regular basis. She also used a lot of lard and double cream, but that's another story.

Bone broth is a prime example of how we lost touch with basic recipes and food lessons from our ancestors. There is nothing basic or banal about a good stock from a flavour or gut perspective. Boiling the bones releases nutrients such as glutamine, collagen, glycine and gelatin that support the health of connective tissue in the body, including that of the gut barrier. As you will have gathered by now, maintaining a healthy gut barrier is important in managing inflammation. Bone broth may also directly contribute to better mood, as glycine can promote a calmer mental state and decrease anxiety – soothing for the soul, it seems, as well as the gut. Homemade broth is really simple to make as you'll see in my recipe on page 205. After roasting and eating an organic chicken, save the bones – that's real nose-to-tail eating. Add it as a base for soups, meat or veg broths, stews or casseroles, or drink it on its own. If you are buying it, ensure that you source organic. While I'm not suggesting that bone broth is some kind of gut health panacea, no single food is, like many proverbs 'chicken soup for the soul' may have some merit after all.

that ferment dairy products, such as yogurt, cheese and milk kefir, eat lactose – the main sugar in milk – so trying to use these in a water kefir would essentially starve them of their food source and your attempt at fermentation would be rather futile. On the flip side, putting water kefir and kombucha cultures into milk would result in a dud ferment, as the microbes you need for this feed on water with sugar. And in the case of vegetables such as sauerkraut it is the sugar in the cabbage leaves that give the microbes the food they need.

Once you've got the combination right, it is about providing a cosy place for them to do their job. Microbes generally prefer a warm temperature to ferment. If you are fermenting in the winter months then make good use of your airing cupboard – we used to find many a jar of 'kraut lurking in various hot spots around our house when we were little, as Dad would gear up to make another batch of his Bigos stew.

the benefits of ferments

Some would say that the benefits of eating fermented foods is based on anecdotal hearsay, but this stuff has been eaten the world over for millennia, notably for its health benefits. As research gains further traction, it is revealing some very exciting and more tangible plus points to including fermented foods regularly in the diet. It is a beautiful demonstration of a longstanding give-and-take relationship, in that we feed microbes with their preferred food and they generously reciprocate. This includes producing compounds such as organic acids that can help with supporting energy, detoxification and the production of neurotransmitter chemicals that have benefits for both gut and brain.

Fermented foods are also higher in both concentration and bioavailability of (the ability for us to best absorb) certain vitamins and minerals, including vitamin B12, biotin, folic acid, calcium, magnesium, potassium and zinc. The fermentation process means that proteins are, to varying degrees, 'pre-digested', and this extends to proteins such as casein in milk products and gluten in bread, which can make them altogether easier to digest and better absorbed. That's why fermented dairy can often be better tolerated over straight-up milk, and why breads such as sourdough can be easier to digest than non-fermented breads. Fermented foods also contain prebiotics, as mentioned earlier, which have a feeding effect on our resident intestinal microbiome.

The stark reality is that a large proportion of us are not eating enough plant-based foods or a varied enough selection.

Furthermore, phytic acid, and other nutrient 'inhibitors' that are naturally present in plant-based foods – like pulses, legumes and grains – and which can affect absorption of minerals such as iron, zinc and calcium are almost negated when they are fermented. These nutrient inhibitors, which are the plants' natural defence mechanism, are designed to irritate the intestinal barrier, another reason why fermenting these plant foods to break down these defences is better for you and your gut.

The other and most obvious benefit of eating fermented foods is ingesting a high number and direct source of microbes that are believed to be beneficial for our gut. Like a 'probiotic' in food form. In addition, fermentation increases lactic acid production, which makes it tricky for many other microbes to thrive, therefore the beneficial acidic-loving bugs win out. It's a quid pro quo then for our resident gut microbiome.

Last but by no means least, there is the extra texture and depth of flavour of fermented foods, which is derived from that natural umami delight they have. Once you foray into fermentation you'll wonder why you didn't start earlier and how the simple addition of a spoonful of 'kraut or kimchi can totally elevate the simplest of sarnies. Check out my Kim-cheese Toastie on page 111 if you need further inspiration for this. You'll find guidance on how to make milk kefir and sauerkraut in my basic recipes section on pages 202 and 199. There are also lots of fermented foods dotted throughout the recipes to give you easy, delicious and practical ways to include more ferments in your diet.

survival of the fittest

The big remaining question is can the microbes in these foods really survive the long and somewhat treacherous journey through the gut once we have eaten them?

If you recall from Chapter 1 they have to get through being chewed and churned, spat at with various acids, enzymes, bile, more enzymes and then find a spot in the large intestine to create a happy home. It sounds like one helluva trek and you wonder how they make it there alive. But survive they do. At least some of them do, and there are strains that seem to be much hardier and more resistant. Furthermore, the beneficial microbes found in fermented foods tend to be the same residents of our own gut microbiome so they positively 'add to the party' so to speak.

soaking, sprouting and activating

Soaking, sprouting and activating grains, legumes, nuts and seeds can assist digestion, enhance the bioavailability of nutrients and help to minimise natural anti-nutrient substances such as phytic acid and saponins that can be irritating to the barrier of the gut. This is of particular relevance for those following an exclusively plant-based diet as it means relying more on these foods to get key nutrients such as protein, iron, calcium and zinc.

To activate grains, legumes, nuts and seeds you will need to soak them overnight in double their volume of filtered water. In the morning, rinse them well before cooking or drying – either in a dehydrator or a very low oven setting for around 10 hours. For those you are cooking, think slow and low just like you would to get tender meat! You can also use spices to boost their digestibility even further – most notably fennel and ginger have calming properties for the stomach. Asafoetida is a herb used in Indian cooking that is said to aid the digestion of beans and legumes. Fermenting beans, in the form of tempeh and miso, also negates some of the anti-nutrients mentioned above. And in grains, something like sourdough would also do the same thing.

Probiotics refers to microbes that are believed to be good for us and the ones that we want to have in our gut. This term should not to be confused with fermented foods. Probiotics refers to supplements, which we'll look at more in the next chapter.

eat the rainbow

Aside from fibre and fermented foods, our microbes love a bit of phytochemical action. Phytochemicals are chemical compounds found in plant-based foods that have antioxidant properties. This means that they have disease-fighting attributes and help to protect the body, including the brain, from free radicals – molecules that can cause inflammation and damage to cells.

Polyphenols are one of the most researched sub-categories of phytochemicals and can be sub-divided into many groups, including lignans (found mainly in seeds and cereal grains); stilbenoids (which include resveratrol, found in the skin of grapes and in peanuts); anthocyanin in berries; glucosinolates (in cruciferous veggies like broccoli, cabbage and cauliflower); carotenoids (in carrots, butternut squash, sweet potatoes and leafy greens); and flavonols, (found in high amounts in tea, coffee, cocoa, dark chocolate and red wine). Yes, a bit of chocolate and a glass of red is good for your gut microbes!

Phytochemicals are basically the pigments that give plants their colour so although 'eating the rainbow' may sound like a cliché it is a great way to make sure you get a broad range of them into your diet. Dress your veggies with cold-pressed extra virgin olive oil and bring in some texture with myriad types of nuts and seeds to give an additional boost of phytochemicals. Another easy addition, to enhance both flavour and polyphenols, is to pack your dishes with herbs and spices, which are abundant in these plant chemicals. Some of those with the highest concentration include turmeric, cinnamon, oregano, thyme, sage, allspice, rosemary and marjoram. Also, you don't always need to use fresh herbs to reap

an apple a day...

The old saying has stood the test of time for good reason. Apples are a great source of pectin, a type of fibre that feeds the microbes in our gut so that they can produce beneficial substances such as SCFAs like butyrate – in fact, butyrate-producing microbes are particularly partial to this type of fibre. And, as we now know, butyrate is crucial for our gut health, as well as helping to manage inflammation more generally, and is related to cognitive health. Apples also provide polyphenol flavonoids that further support the health of the gut microbiome and have systemic protective effects in the body.

To make the pectin more easily accessible to our gut microbes, it's a good idea to stew the apples; stewing releases more of the pectin fibre so the microbes don't have to work so hard to get to it. It's also a really delicious way for us to enjoy apples, particularly when you add spices like cinnamon, allspice and ginger – yet more polyphenols! Check out my Salted Caramel Apples (page 182) or Sherbet Apple Compote (page 95).

the polyphenol benefit as sometimes the dried versions can be even better. Another good tip is opting for the 'wonkier' and organic varieties of fruit and veg as these tend to have a higher phytochemical content and they taste better too. Perfectly imperfect in so many ways.

essential fats

Another vital dietary component for our gut microbiota and brain health are the omega-3 essential fatty acids. The three main types of omega-3 fatty acids are a-linolenic acid (ALA), which is found in plant-based sources such as flaxseed, chia seed and walnuts; eicosapentaenoic acid (EPA); and docosahexaenoic acid (DHA), which are present in oily fish such as salmon, mackerel, sardines and anchovies, organic grass-fed meat and marine algae such as seaweeds. EPA and DHA have a fundamental role in managing inflammation and they form the lipid membrane of every cell in our body, including the myelin sheath that surrounds neurons.

If you only eat plant-based ALA forms of omega-3 it's important to note that the body is pretty poor at converting ALA into EPA and DHA, which are the forms it can utilise. And bear in mind that relying on seaweeds may mean falling short on EPA, as seaweed tends to be higher in DHA; it is also low in fat so you would have to eat a substantial amount to really benefit.

Oily fish are rich in omega-3 and those that are wild typically have higher levels than the farmed versions. Including smaller types of oily fish in your diet, such as sardines, pilchards and anchovies, also means less exposure to metals like mercury, which is a legit concern if you eat a lot of fish like tuna and swordfish. As well as oily fish, omega-3 is present in organic grass-fed meat, organic free-range poultry and in smaller amounts in organic eggs. Not relying solely on one source of omega-3 is a good way to manage this so that we can get a broader intake and meet our requirements for both EPA and DHA.

Including other fats in the diet – organic butter, ghee, coconut (oil, flesh and milk), avocados, nuts and seeds and cold-pressed oils such as extra virgin olive oil – is important for a happier state of mind and gut. Extra virgin olive oil also contains important polyphenols that support our gut microbiota and since our brain is made up of a high percentage of fat, these essential fats help to actively nourish our grey matter.

the lowdown on sugar and food additives

We are all now aware that our diets have changed radically over the past half a century, with increased amounts of unhealthy fats, refined sugar and salt, food additives and artificial sweeteners. While there isn't a huge amount of data to assess the long-term effects of some of these changes, we do know that excessive sugar and fat intake and some of the more widely used additives can promote an overall inflammatory effect in the body, and that this has contributed to a rise in levels of obesity, as well chronic conditions like type-2 diabetes and heart disease. But what does this mean for our gut microbiota and our brain?

sugar

Firstly, let's look at what has become one of the most discussed topics in nutrition: sugar. I think we all know that too much of the stuff

what does 'processed' food really mean?

The term 'processed' in relation to food, generally speaking, has some negative connotations, when actually many foods are processed to some degree or other: olives need to be pressed to make olive oil, butter is churned from the cream of milk, and grapes are pressed and fermented to produce wine. But there is a marked difference between this sort of processing via mechanical methods and the kind that uses heaps of chemicals. When we refer to foods that have been heavily manipulated with artificial ingredients, unnecessary added sugars, unhealthy fats, refined salt and suchlike, this is when the processing results in an end product that is far removed from what our digestive systems and gut microbes would consider food in the true sense of the word. We could call these foods 'ultra-processed'.

Generally, ultra-processed foods are lower in nutritional value and fibre content and often high in refined carbohydrates, sugar and fat. Basically, they are designed for overconsumption and that's why we keep going back for more of them.

What we really need to think about is the source of our foods. Take bread for instance: it is often blamed for various problems, including digestive ailments and weight gain. Bread is a prime example of a food that has been made for millennia, and was probably one of the first 'processed' foods. When it is made in the most traditional way, like a sourdough loaf for instance, it has just two key ingredients, flour and water, which when fermented and baked make the bread more digestible. However, the majority of the bread sold today undergoes a huge amount of chemical processing: the flour is treated and the yeast manipulated to work at speed, with added preservatives to extend shelf life. For the most part (coeliac disease and wheat allergies aside) it is not bread per se that is the 'baddy' but the type of bread we are buying. For many of us the smell of freshly baked bread is the epitome of olfactory nirvana, so why go without when you don't need to?

Realistically, unless you cook everything from scratch, some element of your food is going to be processed, even ultra-processed at times, which is not a bad thing. Just try to juxtapose these foods with home-cooked meals and a diet that is rich in plant foods so that no food is off the menu. Being knowledgeable about our food and where it comes from is empowering but being too strict is not only unnecessary, but also it creates a stressed and anxious mind – and we know already how that affects the health of our gut.

isn't a good thing but having some sugar should be part of a healthy approach to eating and enjoying food. Moreover, sugar forms part of our ancestral eating patterns in the form of fruit and honey, and I truly believe that a decent slice of my mum's amazing blackberry crumble feeds both belly and soul!

Include a wide base of whole foods but don't get hung up trying to achieve the 'perfect' diet, the 'perfect' gut, or the 'perfect' body for that matter.

Enjoying sugar is part of the enjoyment of food. However, the way many of us now consume it is vastly different from when its availability was limited and often seasonal, and our bodies simply haven't caught up. We haven't evolved enough to adapt to this recent and sharp rise in consumption. To give a simple example, an apple contains 30 per cent less sugar (in the form of fructose) than a small (150ml) glass of apple juice. Moreover, because nature perfectly pairs fructose with fibre in the form of an apple, the sugar is absorbed into the bloodstream more slowly than it is from the juice. Aside from causing rapidly fluctuating blood sugar levels that can potentially lead to chronic diseases, most notably type-2 diabetes, and various other health problems, our gut microbes don't like too much fructose as it can cause excessive fermentation, resulting in bloating and gas.

On the other hand, sucrose, as in straight-up white sugar, which is composed of 50 per cent fructose and 50 per cent sucrose, is broken down much higher up in the digestive tract so it doesn't get to the large intestine where most of your gut microbes live. So, contrary to what you may have believed, sucrose doesn't have such a disastrous effect on your gut microbiota. However, excessive consumption of *any* type of sugar still carries with it the chronic disease risks outlined above. That brings me to another important point: the fact that something is a 'natural' sweetener, such as honey, maple syrup, agave or suchlike, doesn't really make much of a difference. Sugar is sugar at the end of the day and it amounts to the same thing.

When we consider the fructose content of one small glass of apple juice, it is easy to see how our overall sugar intake can easily rack up, particularly when the rollercoaster effect they have on our blood sugar encourages us to crave more and more. The food industry has responded to our taste for sweetness by adding sugars into more and more foods – including ones we wouldn't necessarily consider as sweet, such as savoury sauces and condiments.

artificial sweeteners

Many of us have bought into the 'no-added-sugar' story – the idea that artificially sweetened foods and drinks could satisfy our taste for sugar without extra calories and the negative consequences such as weight gain, increase in blood sugars and so on. Sound too good to be true? Then likely it is. Evidence is emerging that links certain artificial sweeteners, including sucralose, aspartame and saccharin, to metabolic diseases like type-2 diabetes. Crucially, they also appear to affect our gut microbiome. Research indicates these fake sugars may alter the metabolic activity of gut microbes and the substances they produce, including butyrate. This gut-derived shift in metabolism can bring with it increased inflammation, which is not good for gut microbial life.

My advice on sugar? A *little* bit of what you fancy does you good. And all things considered, including the gut microbiota, I would go straight-up rather than opt for the artificial stuff. One thing is for sure, we definitely shouldn't feel any guilt around eating sugar, as the self-imposed judgement and anxiety that comes with restriction is far more detrimental than having a bit of cake or chocolate here and there. Ultimately sugar forms part of an overall whole-food and nutrient-dense diet. We just need to be smart about it and enjoy it mindfully and for the treat that it is.

emulsifiers

Another type of food additive we should look at are emulsifiers. You might have assumed that these are found mainly in stereotypical 'junk food' but they pop up in some unexpected places, such as foods in the gluten-free aisles that we might perceive to be 'healthier'. Emulsifiers, which include lecithin, carrageenan, xanthan and guar gum, to name just a few, are there to prevent the separation of ingredients within the product. Emulsifiers can also be used as thickening agents, to improve texture, make products look 'prettier' and extend shelf life. It doesn't sound so bad, does it? But when you look a bit deeper into the effects that some of them can have on our gut it might not be so pretty.

Studies have indicated that certain food emulsifiers can disrupt the gut microbiota by creating a shift in their composition and can even damage the gut barrier. This can allow microbes and other substances to move into the bloodstream, which may lead to more systemic inflammation in the body. And, as we have explored many times already, increased intestinal permeability, or 'leaky gut', and the resulting inflammatory cascade isn't just an issue for our gut, it has significant consequences for the health of our brain. Not all emulsifiers are 'harmful' per se and the idea is not to make you fearful around food. However, cooking from scratch as much as possible will naturally reduce your overall intake of food additives, which I believe to be a good thing.

The key point to consider is the overall quality of your diet, and the *amount* of additives that you are consuming, rather than becoming fixated on avoiding additives altogether. That can be almost impossible to achieve and it doesn't set up a healthy relationship with food in general. It is the cumulative effect of many different additives, along with other mitigating factors, rather than one single cause, that can negatively impact the biome and brain.

for the love of food

Now we have explored the foods to eat to support the health of our gut, and also a couple of caveats to be mindful around, it is important to acknowledge the relationship that we have with our food and nutrition. There are no two ways about it, this is an area that has become extremely confusing, with a cacophony of voices in the mix. It has left a lot of people totally bewildered as to what they 'should' or 'should not' be eating. Restricting entire food groups, labelling foods as 'bad' or 'good' and self-diagnosing intolerances are just some of the ill-informed decisions that have become more common. Unnecessary restriction and elimination of foods can at best leave us with few options on the menu and

feeding mini minds

If we want our little ones to grow up strong and healthy we need to give them a diet that is rich in the nutrients that allow the gut and the brain to thrive. That seems pretty obvious, but kids may not be up for eating much in the way of fermented foods and fibrous veg – pizza and cookies tend to have more appeal. But, as any parent will know, a combination of persuasion and imagination can work wonders.

Start with foods that they already enjoy so that you can put a twist on something that feels familiar, such as my Dad's Spag Bol (page 169). Carrots are a vegetable that many kids will eat without too much fuss. You can double up on fibre by getting them to dip carrot sticks into an avocado dip or hummus and it can be a great snack for them to take to school. Waffles are always fun (at any age!), so try my waffle recipes on pages 94 and 96 – both of them pack in plenty of healthy fibre. Apples, particularly stewed, are great for feeding microbes in the gut (see page 34). Kids usually love stewed apples, particularly if you add in some cinnamon and a drizzle of honey and give them a more enticing name like cinnamon toffee apples or Sherbet Apple Compote (page 95). Sweet potatoes are also brilliant as they are packed full of fibre and antioxidants, and more often than not they suit mini taste buds, especially when made into wedges or fries.

Increasing their intake of food-based sources of beneficial bacteria can mean simply adding in a couple of magic ingredients. This could be swirling a drizzle of honey through a natural full-fat unsweetened 'live' yogurt so that it tastes a bit sweeter on the palate. If your child has an allergy or reacts to dairy then you can use 100 per cent coconut milk yogurt with cultures. Cheese is also an easy sell for a lot of little ones and packs trillions of bacteria into just a small serving – even better if it is unpasteurised. Don't heat the cheese, to ensure maximum microbial benefits, and instead you can (almost) pass off a simple sandwich of grated Cheddar, fresh sourdough bread (another nice gut microbiota feeder) and some sliced tomatoes and maybe a bit of Parmesan, as a riff on a margarita pizza. If they are willing to give sauerkraut a go, try mixing it through cooked vegetables or adding it to a hearty salad or coleslaw to serve with burgers.

Making the plate visually enticing with lots of colours can spark interest so I always encourage parents, where possible, to let kids get their hands in the mix too, so that they can feel proud about eating and enjoying their own creations. My bright and beautiful Rainbow Halloumi Stacks (page 114) might appeal to imaginative kids and, as its name suggests, will add a rainbow of veggies to their plate.

You can also try giving the gut microbiota a nickname (my god-daughter and I call it Bob) and explain to your kids that it is like a pet living inside each of our tummies and it needs feeding with plenty of fibre in the form of vegetables, fruit, grains, nuts and seeds to keep it healthy and happy.

feeling like a bit of a social pariah, but more seriously they can lead to nutritional deficiencies that can have a broader impact on our health. Furthermore, severely limiting entire macro-nutrient food groups such as carbohydrates can reduce our energy levels both mentally and physically. In the case of carbs, when taken to an extreme, this can lead to a gut microbiota that is 'starving', as our microbes need to extract their food predominantly from the fibre that is found in all plant-based carbohydrates. I won't go into the mental side effects when you haven't eaten properly – but there is a reason for the recently coined word 'hangry'.

Note: if you have developed more serious issues with food and your eating patterns you must seek the advice of a professional who can give you the appropriate support.

There should be zero judgement on the decisions that someone takes on what they do or do not want to eat. However, my general advice – unless you have a bona fide diagnosed allergy – is to aim to have a diet that is as inclusive and diverse as possible. Include a wide base of whole foods but don't get hung up trying to achieve the 'perfect' diet, the 'perfect' gut, or the 'perfect' body for that matter – it simply doesn't exist. It is crucial that we get pleasure from our food at the same time as choosing those foods that best support our gut microbiome and our mind.

Once you understand that all foods are available to you, you can enjoy the foods that you might have once thought 'out of bounds' with a sense of balance rather than guilt. When you remove the stigma around 'banned' or 'blamed' foods you will likely feel as though you don't actually want them as much. When we talk about restriction and elimination we are introducing fear and anxiety around eating. By removing these barriers, we also reduce the associated angst, and we know that the physical effects of stress negatively affect the gut as well as our mental wellbeing.

When you go out for a meal with friends or family, make the most of the good company and focus on enjoying the food. This is the time to opt for the dish you *really* want rather than coming to the table with lots of preconceived notions about what you 'should' eat. Stop when you are full: that might mean polishing off the plate, or not. I'd also suggest a nice glass of vin rouge on the side, obviously for the polyphenol benefits!

The concept of eating well, for me anyway, means eating from the soul, with real enjoyment, to gain pleasure and give gratitude. The more that we can be present and focus on the joy of eating the better we will connect to what's on our plate.

Having a healthy, happy and meaningful connection with our food is all about balance, love and respect – if we think of it in that way it will bring us joy from the deepest part of our gut and soul. Food, after all, is more than just a meal. It makes and shapes us biologically, emotionally and, as you now know, is at the heart of our gut microbiota too.

CHAPTER 7

a life less ordinary

IN THE PREVIOUS chapter we explored the foods that can help to nourish our gut microbiota and our mind; now let's look at some of the environmental and lifestyle factors that can affect the microbes in our gut, and their relationship with the brain. After all, eating for the gut and brain is one thing but it is nothing without taking into consideration the way in which the outside world can impact on our internal one.

microbes matter

Most of the microbes that live in our gut are not just harmless but they are also entirely beneficial and necessary for our health and wellbeing. We have evolved together over millennia, yet within the space of three generations our microbes have come under attack as never before. Sometimes we can be more exposed to a relatively small number of potentially pathogenic microbes due to circumstantial shifts in diet, stress or infection but more often than not, our microbes live in perfect harmony with us. It is against their best interest to act aggressively or inappropriately. So why, when we have been working together for some millions of years and for mutually beneficial purposes, would we knowingly then want to destroy them?

The discovery of antibiotics brought about a revolution in the way we treat bacterial infections and, there are no two ways about it, antibiotics are life-saving. However, the use of antibiotics is essentially like a grenade to the gut microbiota, because along with destroying harmful microbes we kill off many of those that protect and support us. This 'blanket bombing' effect can create a huge amount of disarray in the composition of the gut microbiota, which can lead to increased susceptibility to infection, as we have fewer beneficial microbes in our internal army to win out. However, it doesn't take long for microbes to fight back. If you think about it, microbes have developed over billions of years and throughout that time they have seen off many threats. They adapt to survive. So, it's no wonder that the overuse of antibiotics has resulted in the development of antibiotic resistance and so-called superbugs. Basically, the bugs are outwitting us. Darwin's theory of evolution and natural selection – the survival of the fittest – could potentially be coming true in the most frightening of scenarios.

This indiscriminate destruction of our gut microbes can result in a disordered gut microbiota that may have major repercussions for the health of our gut, immune system and gut–brain communication. As we explored in previous chapters, a compromised gut microbiota can result in lower production of the myriad positive substances that play a crucial part in gut–brain communication and managing inflammation, including SCFAs. Fewer of our protective beneficial microbes also makes the gut barrier much more vulnerable, which can lead to 'leaky gut'. This can be especially problematic in infancy, when the immune system and brain circuitry are still developing, and could explain the correlation between early

antibiotic exposure and atopic conditions such as asthma, as well as a possible link with autism (see page 39).

To be clear, I'm not suggesting that antibiotics should not be used. It is more to do with the ubiquitous way that we might take them for things that don't respond to antibiotics, like colds and viruses, or when they're used just as a precautionary or prophylactic method for something that doesn't really seem necessary. We need to think of them as destructive ammo and use them wisely and mindfully.

Antibiotics are not the only medications that can adversely affect our gut health. Other common pills that we pop on a daily basis, such as oral contraceptives and NSAIDs (non-steroidal anti-inflammatories), can shift the composition of the gut microbiota and create damage to the gut barrier. The contraceptive pill can also affect mood, since long-term use depletes nutrients such as B6, which has a vital role in the production of serotonin and GABA – those happy and calming neurotransmitters I described in Chapter 2. And, ironically, we might be taking NSAIDs to reduce inflammation, when in the longer term they actually reduce our overall ability to manage inflammation by weakening the gut barrier.

The fact is we can be too meticulously clean.

Taking umbrage with bacteria and bugs also extends to the cleaning tools that we use in our homes, as well as some of the personal care products we favour. The fact is, we can be too meticulously clean. In a similar way that antibiotics destroy helpful bacteria, the use of lots of antibacterial products can have a deleterious effect on our microbiota. The second largest microbiota after our gut is on our skin, yet we subject it to harsh chemicals. Using more natural cleaning, beauty and personal care products will leave you and your house spick and span rather than sterile.

chemical overload

We are exposed to hundreds of chemicals on a daily basis, not just from food but often unwittingly in myriad environmental ways through the air we breathe, the water we drink, personal-care and household-cleaning products and medications, as mentioned above. While some of these are unavoidable, to a greater or lesser extent, we can have some control over the amount that we are allowing into our personal space. Let's have a look at how this can impact on the health of our gut and our brain…

agriculture and farming

Most of the agricultural crops grown globally, such as fruit, vegetables and grains, are grown with the aid of pesticides. For many farmers,

to supplement or not to supplement?

First things first, we cannot substitute a whole-foods nutrient-dense diet with any kind of supplement. Food comes served up with other bonuses such as fibre and co-factor nutrients that naturally help to enhance absorption of other nutrients. Looking at where we need to fill gaps is really the aim. Gut health is often associated with 'probiotic' supplements. And there are a lot of them out there. So how do we best navigate this and 'sort the men from the boys'?

Before we get into this, the term 'probiotics' refers to microbes that are beneficial for our health and that mostly come from bacteria, although yeast such as *Saccharomyces boulardii* may also pop up in a lot of probiotics.

When choosing a probiotic, firstly we have to check that the microbes in the formula are alive. Different manufacturers will use different methods to deliver these live microbes – either in capsule or liquid form – but they must be able to survive the journey to our large intestine. There also needs to be a considerable number of them in the first place for this reason, as we will invariably lose some along the way during the arduous process of digestion. Aim for at least 1 billion CFU's (which denotes the number of live and active microbes) as the minimum requirement. Another really important point is to check the credentials of the probiotic, by which I mean: are there independent clinical trials and research to back up the claims made by the manufacturer? A bit of patience is also necessary. Probiotics can take a bit of time to take effect, so don't expect an overnight fix. Typically, it can take from 4–12 weeks to see improvements. And probiotics are by no means a 'cure-all' for the gut if you are not working on nourishing your gut microbiome with food that can help it thrive, and managing your stress level.

pesticides are necessary to protect their crops and their livelihoods, but with question marks over the possible negative effects they might have on our own health, and increased awareness of environmental issues, some growers are reducing their pesticide use and moving their farming practice to one that is more sustainable. Of course, not all pesticides are the same but, needless to say, plant foods riddled with pesticides don't have the same levels of phytochemicals that I mentioned in the previous chapter, in comparison to those grown organically. Furthermore, using pesticides to achieve monoculture, uniform crops has also brought a significant loss of diversity and variety in the crops themselves, which is important when we want to aim for diversity in our gut microbiota. You could go as far as to say that *all* nature is connected, and pesticides that affect crops also affect microbes in the soil and have the potential to affect our own gut microbes.

Sourcing organic may also help to reduce some of the more 'toxic' pesticides and is certainly preferable when it comes to meat, poultry, eggs and dairy, as antibiotics can routinely be administered in conventional farming. It also ensures certain standards for the welfare of the animals. However, the reality is that it can be more expensive to buy organic, and when you are feeding an entire family it may not be financially viable, so it's best to pick your battles with this and make organic meat, poultry, eggs and dairy a priority. Also ensure that when buying organic the food has the Soil Association approval stamp – that way you know that the farm has adhered to their high standards.

Buying from local farmers' markets is another good way of getting more transparency about

drastic plastic

I don't think any of us have missed the controversy about the amount of plastic in our rivers and oceans. It has been suggested there is now more plastic than fish in the sea, much of which may take an eternity to degrade. Discarded plastic packaging is literally choking marine life, while microplastics, tiny particles of plastic, have been found in the guts of fish.

There have been indications that microplastics are also popping up in our own poop, which may be affecting our microbial life in the same untoward way that has been demonstrated in studies on fish. It has also been suggested that microplastics may be linked to neurotoxicity, which means they could be affecting the health of the brain. Where possible it is best to try to minimise the use of all plastics. Avoid plastic food packaging, drinks bottles and containers as much as possible. Instead use a glass or steel carry-around bottle, glass or ceramic containers over storing and/or heating food in plastic – and when buying fruit and vegetables, try not to use plastic bags. Mindfully reducing our plastic consumption is something that we all need to be on board with for so many reasons, including the health of our gut microbes.

the methods and/or the chemicals used to grow or make the foods on offer – and meeting the producers brings heightened awareness of and connectivity to our food and the people who grow it. Buying local produce is also better for the environment from the perspective of a reduced carbon footprint and impact on air quality. Sourcing what is seasonally available can also inspire us to try some different veg and fruit – and of course the diversity that brings is great for the gut. It can also be more cost-effective than buying from the supermarket.

sunshine state

Maintaining a sunny disposition is so much easier when the sun is shining – and not just for the obvious reason that it raises our spirits. Vitamin D is a vital nutrient that the body creates when we expose our skin to sunlight, and it is also found in some foods. It is a bit of a misnomer to label it a vitamin because it acts more like a hormone in the body, with a crucial role in maintaining strong and healthy bones, keeping the immune system robust and supporting cardiovascular health. A lack of vitamin D can also affect the composition of our gut microbiota and low levels have also been associated with IBS (irritable bowel syndrome). Furthermore, because vitamin D helps to regulate the release of serotonin, both in the gut and the brain, it has a significant effect on mood.

The fact that most vitamin D is synthesised internally, via skin exposure to sunlight, is great if you live in the sunshine state of California; not so good if, like me, you're a resident of decidedly grey GB. A daily 10 minutes in the sun gives us adequate amounts of vitamin D, but even that can be difficult to achieve at times,

therefore it is important to supplement vitamin D throughout the winter months, unless you are heading off to sunnier climes. Dietary sources of vitamin D include oily fish, eggs and butter, although not in sufficient quantities to meet your daily needs.

microbes like to move

Physical movement is just as important for our mood and mindset as it is for its physical benefits, particularly as some of the endorphin 'feel-good' chemicals that are released when we exercise can improve our outlook immeasurably. This doesn't mean that we need to get carried away with lots of high-intensity exercise like running, spinning and boot-camp classes. Too much of this type of activity over prolonged periods can activate an excessive amount of stress hormones like cortisol and adrenaline, which can leave us feeling flat rather than sprightly, and can negatively affect the health of our gut (see Chapter 4).

We don't have to be a slave to the gym to move our bodies.

It also appears that our gut microbes like to move. Exercise, in moderate amounts, has been shown to positively impact on the composition of the gut microbiota. Furthermore, a simple thing like getting up and walking around can alleviate digestive symptoms such as bloating and gas. Walking is also something most of us can easily build into our daily lives. Getting outdoors gives you the benefits of vitamin D mentioned above – and usually involves more natural movement too. We don't have to slave in the gym to move our bodies, nor is it great to do just an hour of movement and then sit hunched over a computer all day. Rather than thinking that hammering it in the gym will solve everything, we need to move more throughout the day and be mindful of when we've been sitting for too long. Cumulatively this is likely to have a much more positive effect and gives our brain a break from the constant stream of emails and work pressures.

yoga

Yoga is an ancient mindful practice and many of us who have done it will have experienced that deep feeling of calm after some time on the mat. More recently the positive benefits of yoga have been linked to an improvement in many conditions including reducing anxiety, blood pressure and symptoms of gut conditions such as IBS. This is because the breathing techniques intrinsic to the practice itself can help to move us into the 'rest and digest' mode, which has positive effects on the gut–brain connection (see more on this in the box opposite). Flowing through the poses can also have a positive physical impact on the gut and help to alleviate symptoms such as gas, bloating and constipation. The other great thing about yoga is that concentrating on the breathwork and the poses allows us to tune into what we are doing rather than being constantly distracted. You can find plenty of online tutorials, but if you are a novice then it is better to seek out a class to get some personal guidance on the basic positions. It is also another opportunity to engage with others and build crucial personal connections, as well as connecting with yourself.

the art of pooping

When it comes to movement we could extend this to how we best support our bowels to move. Mastering our pooping technique is serious business. Maintaining regularity, as well as satisfaction with our visit to the bathroom, has a lot to do with how we poo. Rushing around and not allowing adequate time to poop does not give our gut ample opportunity to perform at its best. Lots of us have the strongest urge for a bowel movement in the morning, so it is important to let your gut have a bit of 'warm up' time rather than rushing out of the door. Efficiency in our movements is one thing but speed is not what we want to achieve. The prime positioning for pooping can also be tweaked by slightly leaning forward with a straight spine and crucially taking a moment to relax before you begin. Some people find that having a small footstool to elevate the feet, which gives an even better angle, can help further. Whichever way you choose to sit, take a bit of time to relax into your position – although reading material should not be a prerequisite either. Once done, we can take a moment to enjoy a sense of 'evacuation euphoria' and go about our daily business, now that we have done the business.

diaphragmatic 'belly' breathing

Deep breathing forms the basis of many meditative practices, including yoga and t'ai chi, and is believed to support a calm, grounded state both mentally and physically. This is based on the nervous system shift that happens when we engage in such breathing practices, which essentially moves us into 'rest and digest' mode. Diaphragmatic breathing has a stimulating yet soothing effect on the vagus nerve, which passes through the diaphragm and connects to the gut. Stimulating the vagus nerve through diaphragmatic breathing (also called slow abdominal or 'belly' breathing) can immediately lower stress responses and slow heart rate, and also puts the gut into a more restful state.

The great thing with this technique is that you can do it anywhere. Start by breathing through the nose, deep into the abdomen and filling up the lungs from bottom to top until you can't breathe in any more air. Then slowly begin to release the air through the nose until you have fully 'emptied the tank'. You can also use counting to measure the time breathing in and out, to ensure that both parts are of equal measure. A count of four or five is a good number to start with. You can always increase it as you get used to the feeling and the practice. Try this for 5–10 minutes per day at the end of the day to help promote better sleep, to ground yourself in the morning for the day ahead, or whenever you face a stressful situation.

when it's best to rest

In the perpetual stress of the external world we can forget that our bodies and our microbiota need time to simply stop. We will be looking more into mindful practice in the next chapter, but the action of doing nothing and being still has much more gravitas for our mental and physical wellbeing than we might give it credit for. With this, literally, in mind we should take some time every day to be still and check in with ourselves, without judgement or self-criticism. This can be much more challenging than we think but it's necessary. Our modern-day lifestyles can often feel somewhat less than 'ordinary' and overwhelming, so by taking time out to rest, reflect and be present we can find some peace and quiet in what could be perceived as the mundane.

soul food

ONE OF THE biggest challenges to our overall wellbeing, and crucially the gut-brain connection, is our inability to be mindful and present. In the past, the concept of mindfulness was seen by some as a bit 'woo-woo', but it is something that we *all* need to adopt as an integral part of our life. Given the multiple social and external pressures from our technology-driven and media-fuelled lifestyles, is it any wonder we can be addicted to distraction? This, coupled with the fact that we are often disconnected from real people and real life, can impinge on many aspects of our health. Often one of the first areas to show the disgruntled effects of a distracted and disconnected mind is the gut. In this chapter we will be focusing on how nourishing our mind through mindful practice, learning when to disconnect and being more present mentally, is so important for our physical wellbeing and the greater good for our gut health.

eating and being together

The social aspect of eating together is central to mankind's relationship with food. We are naturally social creatures and social interaction, or the lack of it, can have a marked effect on our mental and physical wellbeing. The traditional Mediterranean diet is often held up as an example of a healthy way of eating and it is no coincidence that in Mediterranean culture meals are often eaten with the entire family present. In contrast, our frenetic lifestyles are increasingly solitary and isolated. Families, for example, often eat at scattered times and totally different meals, with little time for conversation. The physical effects of this 'disconnect' are becoming more pronounced and are being reflected in the increase in stress, mood disorders and gut-related conditions – essentially because both our mind and our gut end up feeling overwhelmed and unsatisfied. But we can change this: using mealtimes to sit and talk with the family; by finding joy in meeting and sharing meals with friends; and in time spent with those we truly love.

The effect of loneliness should never be underestimated and has been cited as one of the key drivers in mood disorders, as well as having a detrimental effect on ageing and mortality.

screen survival

The excessive use of digital devices can affect both our gut and brain by increasing the production of stress hormones and reducing the time the body can rest and digest, relax and repair. But it might also be physiologically altering the way in which we use certain areas of the brain.

Some experts reckon that our increased reliance on smartphones, search engines and social media means that we are not using certain parts of our brain as we used to, particularly those related to recall and analytical processing. Search engines give us the answers we are looking for without any effort, but without 'exercise' our analytical prowess can weaken.

In contrast, digital interaction can stimulate certain parts of the brain. MRI scans have shown that activity in the reward centre of our brain and production of dopamine is increased during social media engagement, especially when it is focused on oneself, so you might feel a physiological reward when talking about yourself, more so if you have an audience that is liking what you are saying or posting. You can see how that might play out as a really unhealthy pattern in relationships and the ability to relate to real people takes second place to projecting a digital persona. We might be reducing not just the numbers and quality of gut microbes in our life by being overly stressed and stimulated, but also potentially the amount of meaningful relationships. And that's a lose–lose situation for you and your gut microbiota.

With that in mind, adopting some screen survival techniques can help you to better manage this. Useful tips might be saving a drawer or box in which to put phones away at mealtimes; dedicating a day, or even half a day, per week to leaving the phone off or at home; and going through your social media feeds to consciously unfollow people and accounts that don't nourish you mentally and/or emotionally.

Whenever possible, make it a priority to set aside times to eat together as a family and/or with friends, without external distractions – that means switching off devices that drain our energy and our ability to be present with the people in our lives. Cook together, eat together and even consider the washing up as a team effort. And don't forget the importance of laughter. As the novelist Thomas Mann said, 'laughter is a sunbeam of the soul' and sometimes we forget just how positive a good chuckle with others can be. Laughter can even stimulate the release of 'feel-good' endorphins. Laugh and the whole world, including your gut, laughs with you.

sit and savour

As well as sharing our mealtimes in an enjoyable, relaxed manner, it is important to really connect with and savour our food, even when we are dining alone. Connecting with what's on our plate sounds pretty straightforward, but many of us find it a totally alien concept. Much of this disconnection has been born out of the phenomena of quick, cheap and easily available food. Why bother cooking when you can just pop to the shop, pick up the phone or click on an app and buy something without having to do anything except put it on a plate?

Nowadays we don't even need to step into our kitchens to have a meal ready and waiting. Apps and delivery services mean that with just a few clicks, taps and swipes we can have food at our fingertips 24/7. You might be thinking: *What is wrong with that?* And sure, I'm not suggesting there is anything wrong per se. It can be a really convenient way of helping us to manage our busy lives. However, with this type of 'digital dining' we forgo the actual process of making a meal.

Time is often cited as an issue but the reality is that as soon as we have wolfed down said meal it is often a case of getting back to watching TV, scrolling on devices or working on our phones or laptops. We do have time; we just need to spend it differently. After all, food can be both healthy and fast. A simple bowl of soup, for example, is one of the most nourishing, quick and soul-warming dishes we can make. And sure, cooking food may not seem that appealing to everyone but I would argue that it's more do to with lack of confidence in the kitchen and/or a lack of inspiration, so hopefully my recipes will help: they are all simple to make and offer plenty of ideas for everyday meals. Moreover, most people feel a real sense of achievement in making a meal, as well as a greater appreciation and enjoyment of the food in front of them.

Take the time to chew and taste thoughtfully, truly engaging with your food, valuing these moments and giving your mind a bit of respite.

The very act of cooking also engages the mind in something that isn't about work or other worries. And when you do sit down to eat, why not take the time to chew and taste thoughtfully, truly engaging with your food, valuing these moments and giving your mind a bit of respite? If we are really honest, too few of us take the time to do that.

make every meal a dinner date

Neurogastronomy, a term coined by neuroscientist Gordon M. Shepherd, is an interdisciplinary meeting of neuroscience and psychology. This is a field that studies the link between our perception of food flavours and how that affects our cognitive processing, memory and connection with our food. In essence it is the 'brain on flavour', and relates to the way we use senses such as smell, sounds and sights, in addition to taste, when we are embarking on a meal.

Strange as it may sound, it is unlikely that you would eat a meal and focus purely on the flavours. Just imagine a memory of a really great dinner, everything from the moment you walk in, the heady aromas of dishes being cooked, the ambience and décor of the restaurant, the company you are with, the sounds of wine corks popping and glasses chinking, the way that the food is presented on the plate. All of these contribute to your dining experience, and that's before you have even taken a bite. Then imagine the same meal presented in a takeaway box in a busy queue, while you have minutes to grab your lunch, sitting in front of a computer screen, with a pile of deadlines mounting. The backdrop can have a marked influence on the way that we perceive our meal and how we lock it down in our memory. That's why setting an appropriate 'scene' for every meal is a really important part of connecting with our experience of eating.

Even the very simplest of meals can be transformed into a multi-sensory experience just by framing it more consciously: choosing a nice plate to present your food, rather than eating straight from the packaging; using proper cutlery; selecting a nice napkin; and sitting in an area away from other diversions and distractions, so that you can be fully focused and conscious of your food. It can totally change the mood. And remember, if you are stressed, anxious or in a bad mood then the food isn't going to taste good, even if it is Michelin-starred. Be present with your plate and watch as your senses heighten and your taste buds soar!

bubble-wrapping the mind

Connecting with others and taking time to rest and digest are crucially important for our mental wellbeing. In addition, some kind of daily mindfulness practice can help us to better manage the stresses and strains of modern life. Just like we wouldn't leave the house without our shoes on to protect our feet, we have to think about 'bubble-wrapping' our mind in the same way.

Meditation is at the heart of mindfulness, but this doesn't mean you must follow the stereotypical solitary meditative practice of sitting still and focusing for set periods of time. Some people really engage with this – and the benefits of meditation are proven to be wide-ranging, both psychologically and physically – but don't worry if that's not your thing. Each of us needs to find the type of mindfulness that works for us. Simple guided meditations and apps can be really helpful as they provide a bit of structure and guidance, which can be particularly useful if you are a novice. We know that with regular practice parts of the brain can get stronger: Andy Puddicombe, founder of meditation and mindfulness app Headspace, likens it to when you lift weights in the gym to build muscle. The effect on the gut microbiome is also likely to be very positive, in that the more we can disengage from fight or flight mode the better our chances of achieving a natural state of equilibrium in the gut.

Whether it's yoga, deep breathing (see Diaphragmatic 'Belly' Breathing on page 79) or walking, find what helps your busy mind switch off. Walking is great because it activates similar areas of the brain to those that drive anxiety, therefore if we are engaged in walking it detracts from worrying. This is partly why people often report an immediate release from stress from simply going out for a walk.

mindful not mind full

The extensive amount of choice in our modern world has left many of us confused about what we really need and want. This affects many aspects of our life, but one choice that is required on a daily basis is deciding what to eat. Easier said than done. With such an overwhelming array of foods at our fingertips our decision can be swayed by countless media sources that inform us of the latest 'superfood' or products that will make us slimmer/sexier/fitter. It's all too easy to get swept up in all of this stuff and become fixated on minor details, such as the latest protein powder to put in our morning smoothie or the type of apple cider vinegar we use, when we might not be sleeping well, struggling to have regular bowel movements and stressed out of our head.

If this rings a bell with you, you'll find it much more productive and less stressful to focus on the basics. Avoiding the stream of biased information and removing the pressure to keep up with the latest fad will have a much more positive impact on your mind and gut than any professed 'superfood'. Paring back the amount of time spent on overthinking such matters can open up space for more positive thoughts about your eating and dining habits. You might also apply this to your food purchasing and buy what you need, rather than what you might be cajoled into thinking you need. Buy less and buy better quality to avoid wasting food or money.

Some level of meal planning – not simply thinking about what you will eat for your next meal – is a good idea because, although it takes a little time initially, it can free up your mind for other parts of your life. It can be an enjoyable and cathartic process to write down and see your menu for the week ahead. It also gives focus and clarity to your diet for the week, without being obsessive about it – and you'll avoid having to choose your supper from a supermarket 'grab' or delivery app because you have an empty fridge.

Being more mindful, present and conscious on a daily basis allows us to better tune into what we truly need to be fulfilled and nourished on every level. It can also remind us that we are actually achieving more than we think. It's common to focus on what's *not* going well, an inherent 'negativity bias' that we humans have, but most of us are doing better than we give ourselves credit for. Of course, we can always build on what we have achieved, but focusing on and celebrating what we are doing in the present is far better for both our brains.

mindful eating

You might have heard about the concept of mindful eating. This isn't simply the act of slowing down and chewing thoroughly, although that's certainly part of it. It is about engaging with all of your senses when you are choosing which foods to eat, and during the process of eating, imposing no judgement on what you do, or don't, like to eat and reminding yourself that there are no 'good' or 'bad' foods. It is about knowing that everything is available to you and tuning into what truly nourishes you. Mindful eating is about being more sensitive to the physical sensations of hunger and satiety because this helps to support a better overall relationship with what we eat. Essentially it is learning how to be positive, present and engaged with our food and eating behaviours.

By supporting a more blissful state for our inner microbial life we might just be going some way towards encouraging a mind that is happy and healthy too.

So how can we eat more mindfully? Starting with the moment you get hungry, take a bit of time to tune into what you really need, and if indeed you need it at that moment, with no judgement. Listen to what your body is telling you it wants to eat, rather than grabbing something without any thought. When you decide that you are going to eat, evaluate your options and realise that the choice is entirely

yours, without trying to change or judge your thoughts; this might mean going for broccoli one time and having some chocolate another time. Now start to involve other senses as you prepare and eat your food. Even before you begin eating, notice the shapes and colours of the foods on your plate, and, as you take each bite, tune into the texture, taste, aroma and sounds. Focusing our attention in this way is really important so that our gut and the rest of our body can get the most nourishment out of the food. Once you have finished, tune into the true feeling of being pleasantly satiated and to allow the process of rest and digest to proceed, taking a moment to appreciate the meal that you have just eaten.

The concept of mindful eating is nothing new, it is just something that is easily forgotten in the face of a manic lifestyle in which the brain is distracted in so many ways. In cultures around the world that maintain a focus on the importance of food and company at mealtimes, they don't tend to have the same confusion and angst around food that has become so prevalent in our society.

If it's not something you're familiar with, you might find the practice of mindful eating a little odd to start with, but creating new habits and forming new neural connections around eating can begin with the very next meal you sit down to enjoy. And that's really it, essentially knowing how to enjoy, appreciate and feel connected, with our mind and body, to the very sustenance that helps us thrive.

a new way of thinking

As this chapter has demonstrated, nurturing a happy gut and its many microbial residents isn't just about what we are eating. We need to favourably 'feed' the gut microbiota and our mind in more than just the literal sense.

The 13th-century Persian poet Rumi said, 'There is a voice that doesn't use words. Listen.' Once we understand the myriad ways that our gut connects to our brain we might come to realise that this 'voice' is by no means purely philosophical. In fact, that internal chatter and communication is largely determined by some trillions of microbes in the gut and their seismic impact on our thoughts, feelings, mood, taste sensations and decision-making.

We need to embrace and celebrate our own individuality and that very much includes the core uniqueness of our magnificent gut microbiomes and minds, because they are part of what sets each and every one of us apart.

In a new way of thinking about how we can find a more contented existence, perhaps we could take a moment to consider that if our thinking and mindset relies in some greater part on the health and happiness of our gut microbes then the notion of 'gut feeling' becomes much more significant. Through supporting a more blissful state for our inner microbial life we might just be going some way to encouraging a mind that is happy and healthy too.

Something tells me that we should learn to trust and tune into the innate wisdom, instinct and collective 'voice' of our trillions of magical microbes.

part 2

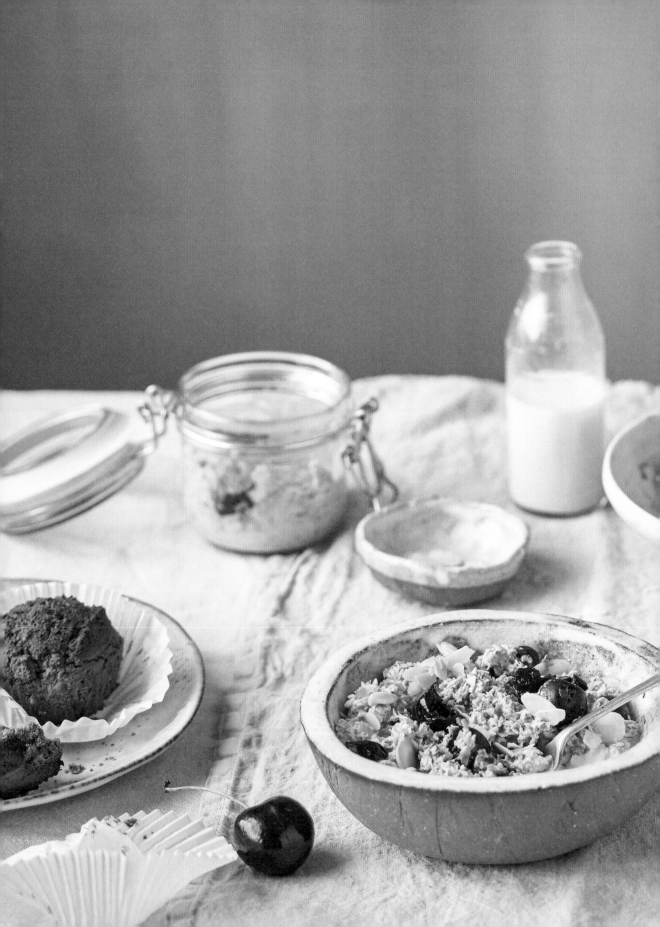

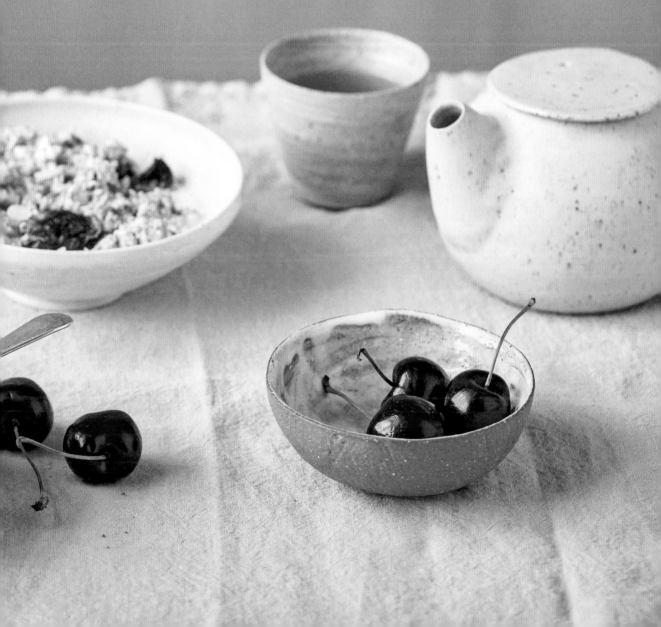

breakfast
and brunch

buckwheat, caraway and pumpkin seed bread

The aroma of this bread baking will create a relaxing olfactory sensation. Buckwheat is naturally gluten free, making this bread ideal if your gut gets a bit stressed by gluten-containing grains. Buckwheat is also rich in B vitamins, which are important for the adrenal glands and brain, plus it provides plentiful amounts of fibre to keep our microbes happy. Pumpkin seeds are one of the highest dietary sources of zinc, a mineral that helps us to manage the effects of stress – and they taste ace in this loaf. This freezes well: slice it before freezing and then simply defrost a slice when needed.

makes 1 loaf

1 tablespoon ground flaxseed

450ml plus 3 tablespoons filtered water

200g buckwheat flour (ideally made from sprouted buckwheat)

100g ground almonds

100g pumpkin seeds

1 tablespoon caraway seeds

2 teaspoons bicarbonate of soda

1 teaspoon sea salt

2 tablespoons apple cider vinegar

In a small bowl, mix the ground flaxseed with 3 tablespoons of filtered water and set aside while you prep the other ingredients.

In a large bowl, mix the buckwheat flour, ground almonds, pumpkin seeds, caraway seeds, bicarbonate of soda and sea salt. Add the apple cider vinegar, 450ml filtered water and the soaked flaxseed and mix well to make a dough. Cover the bowl with a clean tea towel and leave for 1½ hours.

Preheat the oven to 180°C/Gas 4. Line a 900g loaf tin with baking parchment so that it hangs over the long sides of the tin (this will help you remove the bread once it's cooked). Pour the mixture into the loaf tin and bake for 1¼ hours.

Remove from the oven and leave to cool in the tin for 5 minutes. Then, using the baking parchment, carefully lift out the loaf and place on a wire rack to cool completely. Store in the fridge for up to 3 days or slice and freeze.

tip

Grinding your flaxseed from whole fresh seeds is the best way to obtain maximum benefit. Always store your flaxseed in the fridge as it can go rancid quite quickly.

avocado and pea smash

Avocados and peas are both excellent sources of fibre, as well as containing vitamins and minerals that support the adrenal glands, which have a major effect on stress levels. Serve this on sourdough or the buckwheat bread opposite, or use to top baked sweet potato.

serves 2

1 fully ripe avocado
Juice of ½ lemon
50g frozen peas
Small handful fresh parsley, roughly chopped
1 tablespoon extra virgin olive oil
½ teaspoon ground coriander
Generous pinch chilli flakes
Sea salt and black pepper

Remove the flesh from the avocado and mash it in a bowl, using a fork. Add the lemon juice.

Cook the peas in boiling water for 2 minutes. Drain and rinse well with cold water. Mash the peas using a fork, leaving some texture. Add to the avocado.

Add the parsley, olive oil, coriander, chilli flakes, a couple of pinches of salt and a pinch of pepper and mix through. Store in the fridge until ready to serve.

peanut butter and cinnamon overnight oats

This is a really simple and delicious breakfast. Oats have a prebiotic effect, 'feeding' the microbiome, while the yogurt adds a boost of natural bacteria that can help to suppost our gut.

serves 1

50g oats (ideally sprouted)
100ml milk of your choice
1 tablespoon peanut butter
1 teaspoon ground cinnamon
1 teaspoon raw honey, plus extra to serve (optional)
2–3 tablespoons full fat natural yogurt

Put all the ingredients, except the yogurt, into a serving bowl or jar. Mix, cover and leave in the fridge overnight.

In the morning, remove from the fridge and add a couple of tablespoons of yogurt. Drizzle with an extra teaspoon of honey if you like it a bit sweeter.

bakewell bircher

This will have you positively jumping out of bed in the morning. The combination of oats and cherries can support the production of melatonin, which is important for regulating the sleep–wake cycles. In addition, both are an excellent source of fibre for our gut microbes. Almonds supply magnesium, which is key for relaxation, and they also have a rather soothing effect on the palate.

serves 1

2 tablespoons flaked almonds
(see tip)

50g oats (ideally sprouted)

15g frozen unsweetened cherries

½ tablespoon almond butter

½ teaspoon almond extract

75ml unsweetened almond milk
(or milk of your choice), plus extra
if needed

Preheat the oven to 180°C/Gas 4. Line a baking tray with baking parchment. Spread the flaked almonds on the baking tray and bake for 20 minutes. Leave to cool and then store in an airtight container.

Prepare the bircher the night before you want to eat it. Mix all of the ingredients (except the toasted flaked almonds) together in a bowl. Cover and leave in the fridge overnight.

In the morning, remove from the fridge and leave for 10 minutes to come to room temperature. If it has set too thick you may want to add a little more almond milk. Top with the toasted flaked almonds.

tip

When toasting the flaked almonds I suggest you do a bigger batch, as they are lovely sprinkled on top of porridge or yogurt and through salads.

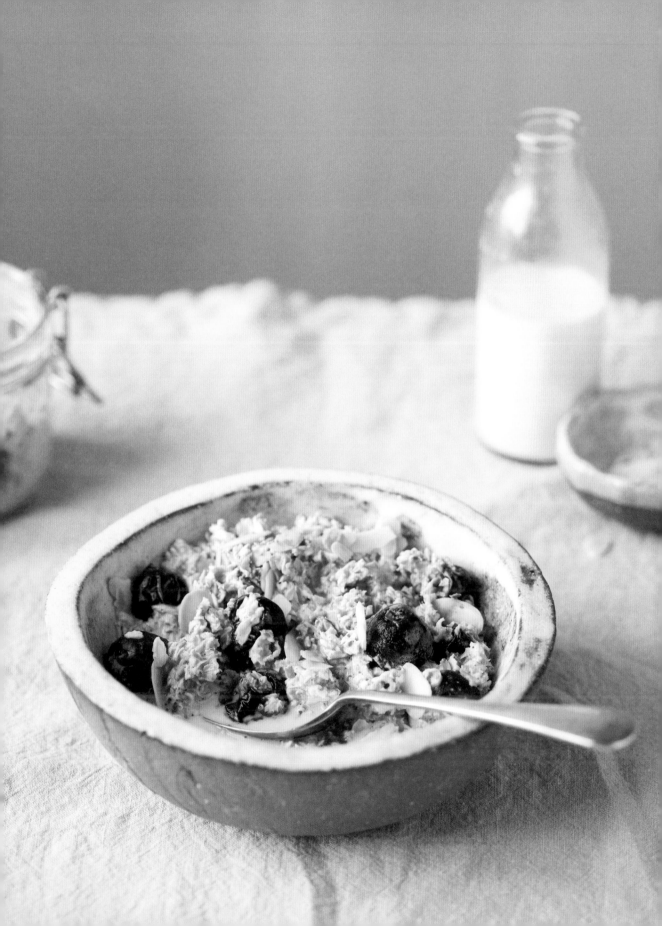

tiger nut waffles

This recipe uses tiger nut flour which is naturally sweet and packed full of resistant starch and fibre that your microbes will love. This is such an easy batter to make and it's a great way to get kids involved in making as well as enjoying their food.

serves 2

150g tiger nut flour or powder
½ teaspoon bicarbonate of soda
½ teaspoon vanilla extract
2 tablespoons apple cider vinegar
200ml unsweetened almond milk or Cashew coconut milk (page xx)
½ teaspoon organic butter or coconut oil for greasing

to serve

Full fat natural yogurt or whipped ricotta

Raw honey to drizzle

Preheat a waffle maker.

Sift the flour into a bowl. Add the bicarbonate of soda and stir through. Add the vanilla extract and apple cider vinegar then slowly add the milk, mixing to create a batter. Let sit for 5 minutes.

Use the butter or coconut oil to grease both the base and the top of the waffle maker: I use a small brush to ensure it is evenly coated. Add the batter to the waffle maker, and cook according to the manufacturer's instructions – this usually takes about 5–10 minutes. Some waffle makers make one waffle at a time, others make two or four waffles, and the size of the waffles varies, so you may need to make the waffles in batches.

Serve with yogurt or whipped ricotta and drizzle with honey.

sherbet apple compote

These stewed apples are given a sherbety twist with the addition of baobab – a citrusy fruit that is rich in micronutrients and high in fibre. This dynamic duo of fruit can help microbes in the gut microbiome to produce substances such as butyrate that support both gut and brain. Use to top porridge. A couple of tablespoons of the compote can also be served with yogurt as a dessert or sweet snack.

makes 2–3 servings

200g apples
Approx. 2 tablespoons filtered water
2 heaped tablespoons baobab powder
1 teaspoon raw honey

Do not peel the apples, just chop them into 5cm cubes, discarding the cores. Place in a large saucepan, add a small amount of filtered water to cover the base of the pan and bring to the boil over a medium heat. Reduce the heat and simmer for 10 minutes.

When the apples are soft, remove from the heat and stir through the baobab powder and honey. Serve warm or store in the fridge in a ceramic or glass container; this will keep for 2–3 days.

cumin scramble and courgette waffles

Inspired by a trip to Marrakech, a city that is bursting with flavours and tantalising taste combinations, I created these waffles. The courgette and coconut flour batter provides fibre that is great for the gut, and it's a nice alternative if you feel that wheat or gluten leaves your digestion a bit 'withered'. Organic eggs provide plenty of key brain and mood nutrients.

serves 2

4 organic eggs
¼ teaspoon ground cumin
Sea salt and black pepper
1 tablespoon organic butter
Extra virgin olive oil to drizzle

courgette waffles

1 small–medium courgette (approx. 150g), shredded or grated
25g coconut flour
3–4 sprigs fresh thyme, leaves picked
2 organic eggs
1 teaspoon organic butter for greasing

Preheat a waffle maker.

To make the waffles, put the courgette in a large bowl then add the coconut flour, most of the thyme leaves (reserve a few to garnish) and the eggs, and season with salt and pepper. Mix to make a thick, dough-like batter. Use the butter to grease both the base and the top of the waffle maker. Spoon the batter into the waffle maker, pressing it in evenly, and cook according to the manufacturer's instructions – this usually takes about 8–10 minutes but check after 5 minutes.

Meanwhile, whisk the eggs with the cumin and a pinch of black pepper and sea salt. Melt the butter in a saucepan over a very low heat, add the eggs and cook very gently, stirring regularly, until cooked to your liking.

Once the waffles are done, put one on each plate. Top with the scrambled eggs, a generous pinch of sea salt and a grinding of black pepper, a drizzle of olive oil and a sprinkling of thyme leaves.

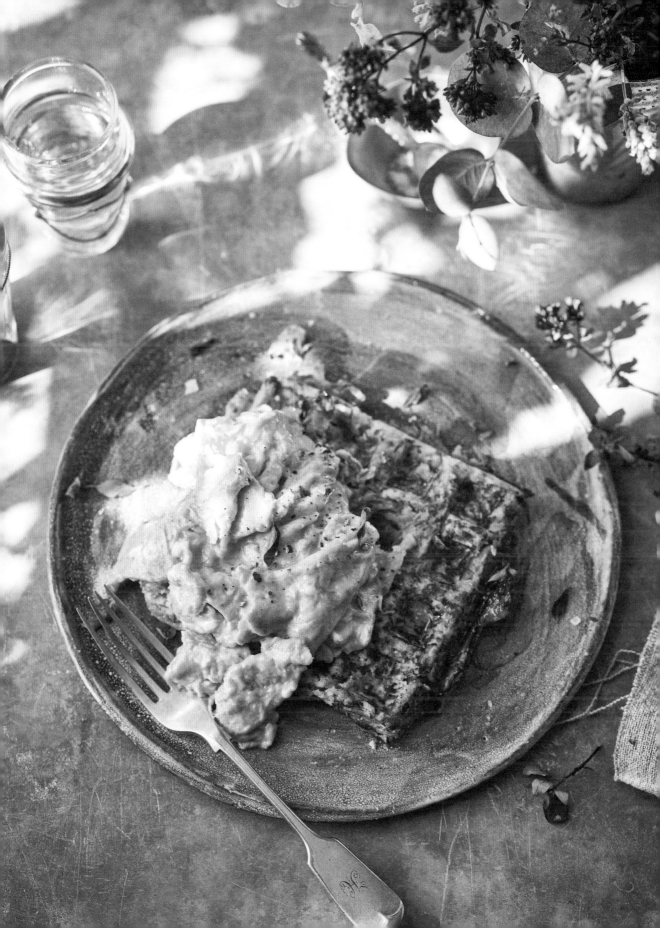

pecan pie granola

Start your day well with this heavenly granola that evokes everything glorious about a sumptuous pecan pie. Oats are an excellent source of beta-glucan fibre, which is widely recognised as having cholesterol-lowering properties, but less well-known is the fact that they help 'feed' the microbiome. You can double the ingredients to make more, as this is sure to be a big hit. Kids in particular will love it – watch their eyes light up as the toasty aromas fill your kitchen. Serve with yogurt or milk and fresh berries or a spoonful of stewed apple.

makes 6–8 servings

125g pecans, roughly chopped

25g coconut chips

75g flaked almonds

100g oats (ideally sprouted)

1 teaspoon ground cinnamon

¼ teaspoon sea salt

100ml maple syrup

1 teaspoon vanilla extract

15g organic butter, melted (or 1 tablespoon coconut oil for a vegan version)

Preheat the oven to 150°C/Gas 2. Line a baking tray with baking parchment.

Combine all the dry ingredients in a large bowl and mix. Add the maple syrup, vanilla and melted butter and combine thoroughly. Spread the mixture over the baking tray and bake for 40–45 minutes until golden.

Leave until cold, then break into smaller chunks. Store in an airtight glass or ceramic container for up to 1 month.

portobello egg 'muffins'

A brilliant and super-quick brunch that anyone can master, this satisfying recipe is a great way to regain that core connection with our food. It uses portobello mushrooms as the 'bun', which provides a source of prebiotics to feed the microbiome and is also a good option for those who cannot tolerate wheat. Eggs are like little multivitamins: their exceptional nutritional value has benefits for both brain and gut.

serves 2

4 large portobello mushroom caps
4 organic eggs
2 handfuls baby spinach leaves
Sea salt and black pepper
Extra virgin olive oil to drizzle

Preheat the grill to medium. Clean the mushrooms and season with salt and pepper. Place in the grill pan, cap side down, and grill for around 10 minutes, or until cooked through.

Meanwhile, bring a large saucepan of water to the boil.

Crack the eggs into individual ramekins or very small bowls. Once the water has boiled, take the pan off the heat and turn the heat down to low. Gently drop the eggs into the water and put the pan back over the heat for 2½ minutes: use a timer for this.

Your mushrooms should be done by now so pop them on the serving plates. Then carefully lift the eggs out of the water and onto a piece of kitchen paper to drain briefly. Put the spinach leaves on top of the mushrooms and then place one egg on each mushroom. Drizzle with olive oil and add a few generous pinches of salt.

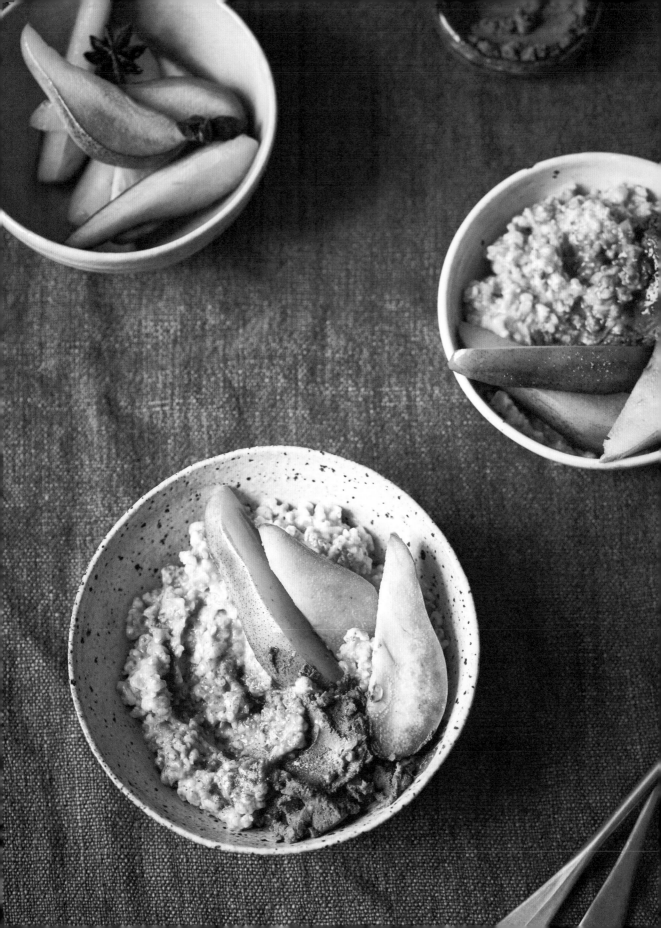

chestnut porridge, star anise pears and chestnut cocoa cream

A nourishing and hearty start to the day. Oats and chestnut flour provide a duo of fibre to support the microbiome. The pears introduce another source of fuel for our microbes and the cocoa cream provides an additional boost of antioxidants, so it's great for our gut as well as giving us something to smile about.

serves 2

2 pears
2 star anise

chestnut porridge

100g oats (ideally sprouted)
2 tablespoons chestnut flour
400ml filtered water
1 teaspoon vanilla extract or seeds from 1 vanilla pod

chestnut and cocoa cream

2 tablespoons coconut butter
3 tablespoons chestnut purée
3 tablespoons chestnut flour
2 tablespoons unsweetened cocoa powder
50ml filtered water

First make the chestnut and cocoa cream. Put the coconut butter in a small bowl and beat to soften slightly. Add the remaining ingredients and beat to a creamy consistency. Place in the fridge to chill.

Cut the pears into eighths, cutting out and discarding the seeds. Place in a large saucepan, adding a small amount of filtered water to cover the base of the pan by about 1cm. Add the star anise. Bring to the boil then reduce the heat, cover the pan and simmer for 10 minutes. Using a slotted spoon, lift out the pears and place on a plate. Remove the star anise, leave to dry and save for another batch.

To make the porridge, place all the ingredients in a saucepan and mix well. Bring to the boil then reduce the heat and simmer for about 10 minutes, stirring occasionally.

Divide the porridge between two bowls and serve with a spoonful of the chestnut cream and the sliced pears.

fig, honey and almond oat bakes

These oaty bakes are all about the satisfaction factor – they taste great, they'll keep the microbes in your gut happy and are comforting too. The figs, oats and almonds provide a diversity of fibre and the honey gives a balanced flavour. They are great for breakfast with a dollop of crème fraîche or coconut yogurt and they freeze well too.

makes 16 squares

150g dried figs, roughly chopped
300g oats (ideally sprouted)
40g flaked almonds
¼ teaspoon sea salt
100g raw honey
2 tablespoons almond butter
½ teaspoon vanilla extract
200ml unsweetened oat milk
organic butter for greasing

Preheat the oven to 190°C/Gas 5. Butter a 15cm square baking tin.

Put the figs into a food processor and pulse to break up into smaller chunks. Add the oats, almonds and salt and pulse for another 30 seconds. Then add the honey, almond butter, vanilla and oat milk and pulse until well mixed. Spoon the mixture into the baking tin, spread evenly and bake for 30 minutes.

Remove from the oven and leave in the tin to cool completely. Cut into 16 pieces and store in an airtight glass or ceramic container in the fridge for up to 3–4 days.

coffee and walnut loaf

Coffee and walnut is a classic flavour combination that makes this delicious loaf perfect for breakfast or a mid-morning snack. As well as coffee extract, I've used ground chicory to enhance the flavour. Chicory is a prebiotic so it can have added benefits for our gut health. I've used a base of tiger nut flour: this is naturally sweet and is an excellent source of resistant starch and fibre that helps to boost our microbiome and in turn encourage a happier start to the day.

makes 1 loaf (approx. 12 slices)

250g tiger nut flour
85g walnuts
10g ground chicory
½ teaspoon bicarbonate of soda
1 tablespoon coconut butter
1 teaspoon raw honey
1 tablespoon apple cider vinegar
3 teaspoons coffee extract
½ teaspoon vanilla extract
150ml filtered water

Preheat the oven to 180°C/Gas 4. Line a small (450g) loaf tin with baking parchment so that it hangs over the long sides of the tin (this will help you remove the loaf once it's cooked).

Place the tiger nut flour, walnuts, chicory and bicarbonate of soda into a food processor and pulse briefly to combine. Then add the coconut butter, honey, apple cider vinegar, coffee and vanilla extracts and water. Pulse again until you have a thick dough. Transfer to the loaf tin and bake for 45 minutes.

Remove from the oven and use the baking parchment to lift the loaf out of the tin and onto a wire rack. After around 5 minutes, carefully remove the baking paper and leave to cool fully. Store in the fridge for up to 3 days or slice and freeze.

peanut and miso muffins

Peanut and miso are a match made in muffin heaven! These muffins have a base of fibre-rich tiger nut flour that can help to make our microbes altogether cheerier. Great for breakfast served with yogurt on the side, or to take to work or pack into lunchboxes. Die-hard PB fans can serve with an extra slick of peanut butter!

makes 6 muffins

250g tiger nut flour
½ teaspoon bicarbonate of soda
80g crunchy peanut butter
1 tablespoon unpasteurised miso paste
½ teaspoon vanilla extract
1 tablespoon apple cider vinegar
100ml filtered water

Preheat the oven to 200°C/Gas 6. Place six large paper muffin cases in a muffin tin.

Put the flour and bicarbonate of soda into a food processor and pulse for 30 seconds to combine and break up any lumps in the flour. Add the peanut butter, miso paste, vanilla and apple cider vinegar and pulse to combine. Then gradually add the water to make a thick batter.

Using an ice cream scoop, add one generous scoop of the batter into each of the muffin cases. Bake for 25 minutes.

Leave to cool in the tin for 5 minutes and then transfer to a wire rack to cool completely. Store in an airtight container for up to 2–3 days.

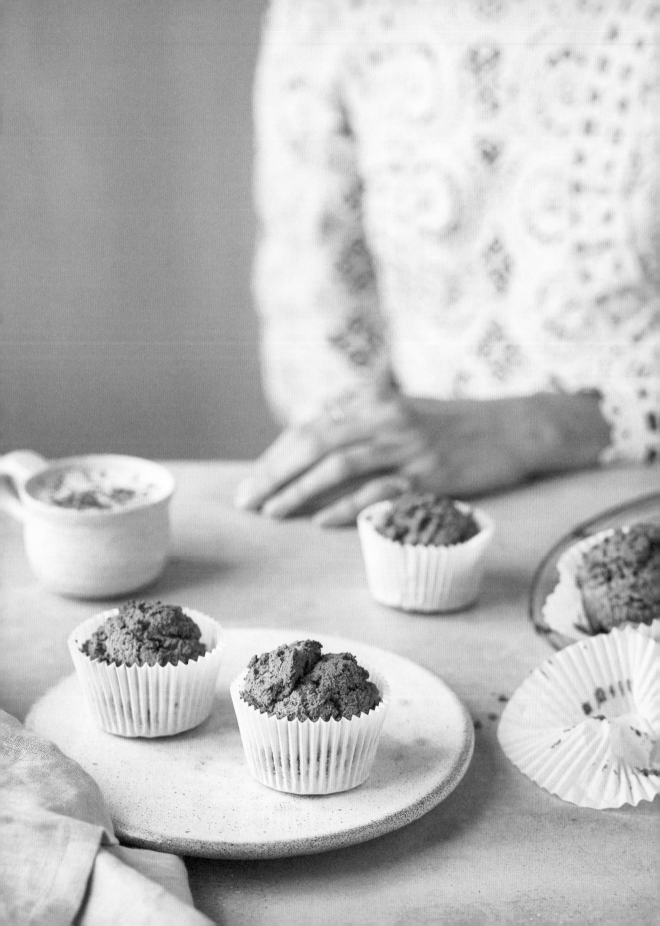

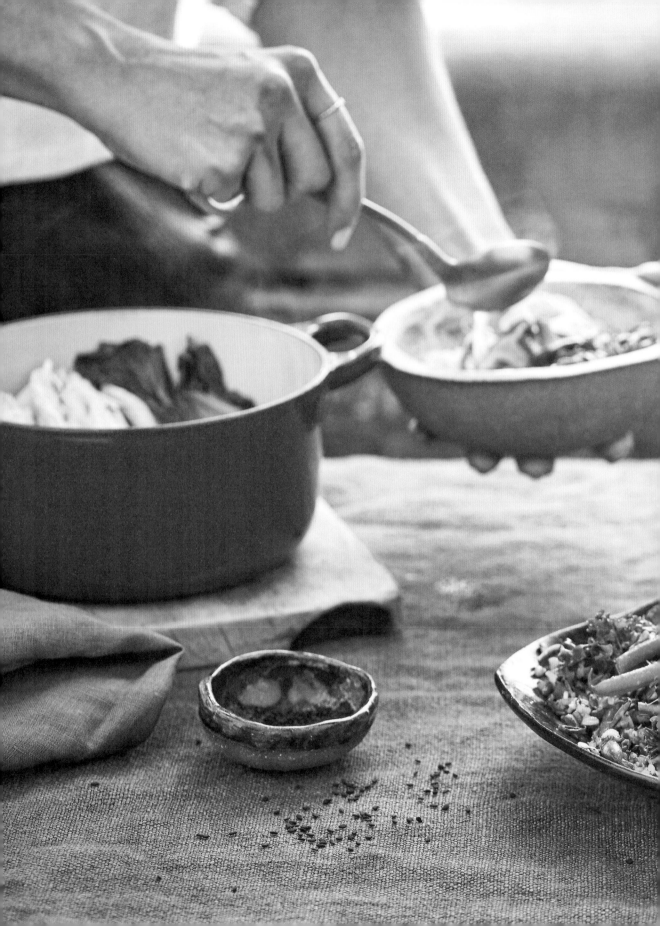

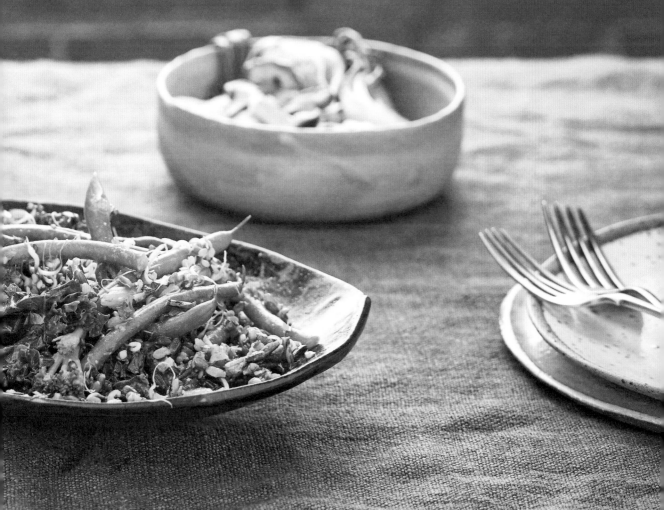

soups, salads
and light meals

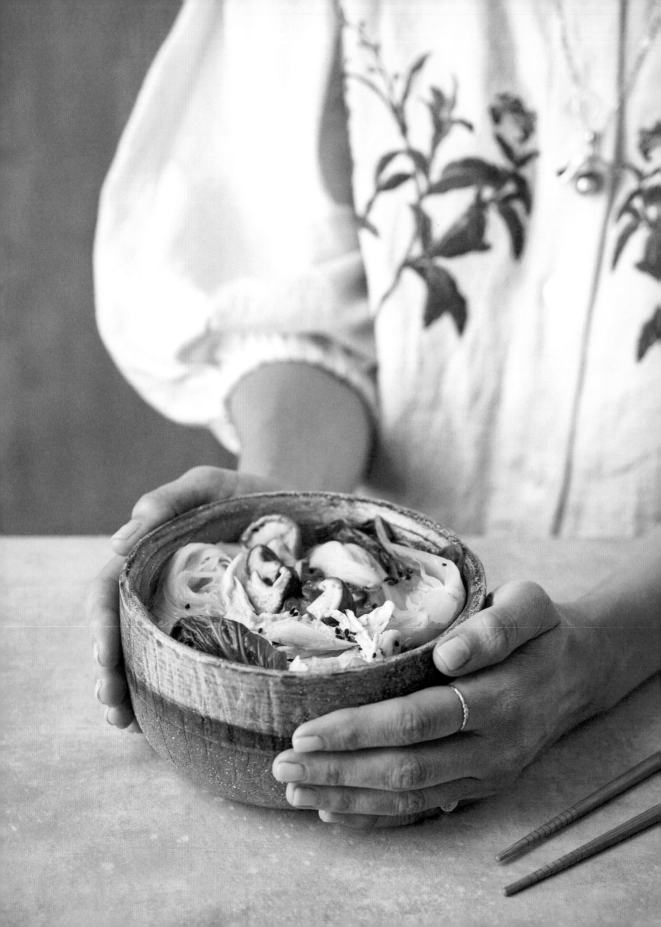

sesame and ginger chicken noodle soup

Chicken soup is said to be good for the soul, so this recipe is designed to provide some heartfelt nourishment for your mind as well as your microbiome. Bone broth contains amino acids that support the barrier of the gut and may help to manage inflammation. Spicy ginger is a natural anti-inflammatory and the gentle heat of this soup really does warm the soul and the belly.

serves 2

1 litre organic chicken bone broth

2–3cm piece of fresh ginger, peeled and finely sliced

1 garlic clove, crushed

2 organic free range chicken breasts

100g rice noodles

100g fresh shiitake mushrooms, sliced

120g pak choi, halved

2 teaspoons tamari

2 teaspoons mirin

Sesame oil to drizzle

1 teaspoon black sesame seeds

Heat the broth in a saucepan, add the ginger and garlic and bring to the boil. Turn down the heat to a gentle simmer, add the chicken breasts and simmer for about 10 minutes until the chicken is cooked through.

Remove the chicken from the pan and place on a chopping board. Add the noodles to the broth, turn up the heat and cook for 5 minutes. Add the mushrooms and pak choi, tamari and mirin and cook for a further 3–4 minutes.

Meanwhile, shred the chicken. Put it back into the broth and heat through for a minute, stirring. Ladle into bowls, drizzle with a little sesame oil and sprinkle with the sesame seeds.

hap-pea soup

This vibrant green soup is a joy to the eyes and the taste buds and, if you have kids, is a great way to get them to enjoy more veggies. Peas, leeks and spinach are full of fibre, vitamins and minerals that support the microbiome and the mind. The bone broth can also soothe the gut and gives an extra boost of flavour. Serve with fresh sourdough, generously smeared with butter.

serves 2

1 tablespoon organic butter
2 leeks, finely sliced
350ml organic chicken bone broth
250g frozen peas
100g fresh spinach leaves
50g ricotta
Generous handful fresh mint leaves
100ml filtered water
Sea salt

Melt the butter in a large saucepan over a medium heat. Add the leeks and stir to coat in the butter. Add the broth and peas and simmer for 5 minutes. Add the spinach and cook for another minute until wilted.

Pour the mixture into a blender. Add the ricotta, mint, the water and a pinch of sea salt and blend until smooth.

You shouldn't need to reheat if eating immediately, but if necessary, pop the soup back into the saucepan and gently heat through before serving.

kim-cheese toastie

Who doesn't love a cheese toastie? Adding the cheese *after* toasting the bread means that you max on the beneficial bacteria naturally present in the cheese and kimchi, as most of them are destroyed by heating. Sourdough provides an extra boost of fibre for our microbes to enjoy. Joyfully easy and tasty!

serves 2

4 slices sourdough bread
1 pat organic butter
75g unpasteurised Manchego cheese, cut into thin slices
4 tablespoons kimchi

Toast the sourdough on both sides. Spread with the butter. Lay the cheese on two slices of the toast, top with the kimchi and the second slice of toast. Cut diagonally into triangles.

tarragon tapenade

This tapenade is super easy to make and it is brimming with antioxidants and healthy oils. The olives and olive oil are a rich source of oleic acid that can help to manage inflammation, supporting the microbiome and the functioning of the brain. It tastes great spread on toasted sourdough and topped with sliced tomatoes or a poached egg. It's also perfect as a dip with vegetable crudités.

makes approx. 200g

45g flaked almonds
1 bunch fresh tarragon, chopped
180g pitted olives
4 tablespoons extra virgin olive oil
1 small garlic clove, crushed (or ¼ teaspoon garlic powder)
½ teaspoon onion powder
1 teaspoon fennel seeds
2 tablespoons drained capers
Juice of 1 lemon
Pinch sea salt and black pepper

Preheat the oven to 150°C/Gas 2. Line a baking tray with baking parchment. Spread the flaked almonds on the baking tray and bake for 20 minutes. Remove from the oven and leave to cool slightly.

Add the almonds and all of the other ingredients to a food processor and pulse to create a thick spread – I like to keep some texture but you may prefer it smoother. You will need to stop and scrape from time to time. Transfer to a container and store in the fridge for up to 5 days.

sourdough, ricotta, figs and nigella

This is a brilliant lunch dish – simple, sumptuous and satisfying. Ricotta is an Italian soft cheese that is made from the whey left over from producing other cheeses. If you find that casein (found in most cheeses) creates 'disturbance' in your gut, ricotta may give a much more favourable response. It is a good source of tryptophan, an essential amino acid that aids the production of hormones that regulate the sleep–wake cycle. Figs and sourdough are good sources of magnesium, a mineral that also helps with sleep.

serves 2

2 large slices sourdough bread
100g ricotta
2 or 3 fresh figs, sliced
1 teaspoon nigella seeds
Raw honey to drizzle

Toast the sourdough. Spread with the ricotta and lay the sliced figs on top. Scatter over the nigella seeds and drizzle with honey. That's it!

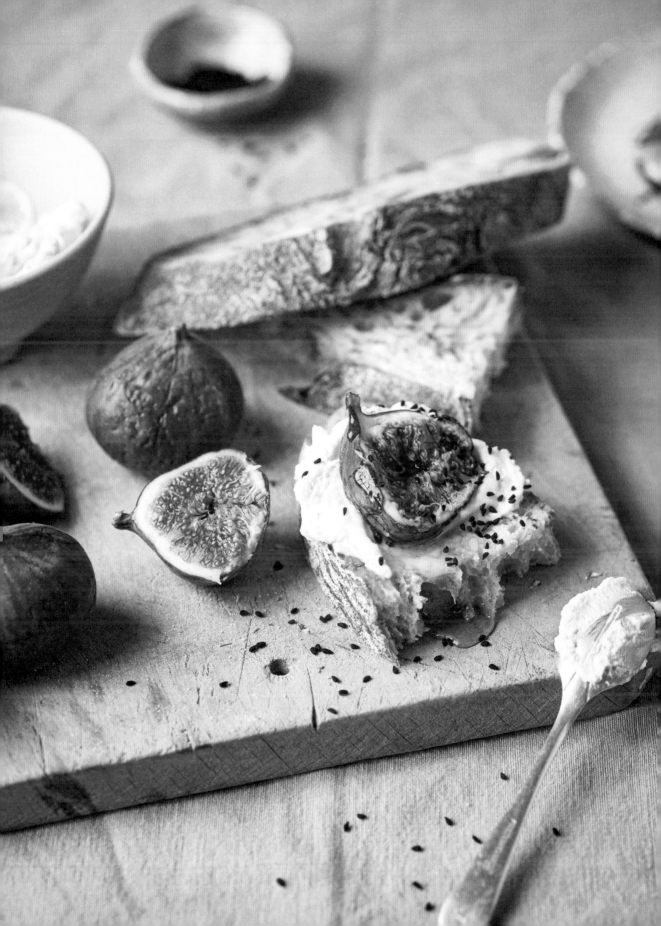

rainbow halloumi stacks

This epitomises the fun that can be had with food. It's playful, delicious and as well as giving our eyes and mind a treat, the rainbow of veggies provides great fibre for our microbiome.

makes 4 stacks (1–2 stacks per person)

1 large beetroot, unpeeled

1 butternut squash, peeled

1 aubergine

1 yellow pepper

2 tablespoons organic butter, melted

1 large red beef tomato

1 avocado

Squeeze lemon juice

200g halloumi, cut into 1cm thick slices

Small handful baby spinach leaves (around 5–6 leaves per stack)

Sea salt

Extra virgin olive oil to drizzle

First, steam or boil your beetroot for 40–45 minutes until tender. Drain and leave to cool.

Preheat the oven to 200°C/Gas 6. Line two baking trays with baking parchment.

You will need four slices of each vegetable (one per stack). Slice the smaller end (the one without seeds) of the butternut squash into discs about 1cm thick. Lay them on a baking tray. Slice the aubergine into discs about 2–3cm thick and put these on the baking tray. Slice off the top (stalk end) of the yellow pepper and remove the seeds. Slice into rings, about 2–3cm thick, and place on the baking tray. Drizzle the butter evenly over the veggies and add a generous sprinkling of sea salt. Put the trays in the oven and roast for 15 minutes.

Meanwhile, peel the beetroot and slice it into 1cm thick slices. After 15 minutes, turn the vegetables over, add the beetroot slices and roast for a further 15 minutes

Cut the tomato into 1cm thick slices. Cut the avocado in half, take out the stone, scoop out the flesh and mash with a fork, adding a squeeze of lemon juice and a pinch of sea salt.

Once the veggies are cooked, remove from the oven and leave to cool.

Preheat the grill to medium. Grill the halloumi for 2–3 minutes on each side until nicely browned.

To assemble the stacks, start with a slice of squash, then tomato, next the pepper, then a few baby spinach leaves with a quarter of the avocado mash on top, next the aubergine, then the beetroot and finally the halloumi. Season each stack with a generous pinch of sea salt and drizzle with olive oil.

lentil, tomato and walnut poached egg salad

This hearty warm salad includes three tryptophan-rich foods: lentils, walnuts and eggs. Tryptophan is the precursor to serotonin, which helps support a happier mood in mind and gut. The recipe also contains spinach to provide a boost of vitamins and minerals to assist with this. A super easy dish for lunch or a light supper.

serves 2

200g Puy lentils, preferably soaked for 7 hours, then rinsed

2 organic eggs

Extra virgin olive oil for frying

50g cherry tomatoes, halved

2 handfuls spinach leaves

2 teaspoons apple cider vinegar

3–4 walnuts, lightly crushed

Sea salt

Cook the lentils in boiling water for 30–40 minutes until tender. Drain, rinse and set to one side.

Bring a large saucepan of water to the boil.

Crack the eggs into individual ramekins or very small bowls. Once the water has boiled take the pan off the heat and reduce the heat to low. Drop the eggs into the water and put back on the heat for 2½ minutes: use a timer for this.

Meanwhile, heat a little olive oil in a large frying pan over a low heat. Add the cooked lentils, tomatoes and spinach and warm through for a couple of minutes. Take off the heat, add the apple cider vinegar and mix through.

Divide the lentil mix between two serving plates. Your eggs should be done by now, so gently remove from the hot water and place on a piece of kitchen paper to drain briefly, then place on top of the lentils. Sprinkle over the walnuts, a couple of generous pinches of sea salt and a drizzle of olive oil.

greens and grains with a miso mustard dressing

This bountiful bowl of rice, veggies, nuts and seeds provides a feast of fibre and antioxidants for the many microbes in our gut, helping them to produce substances that play a part in managing inflammation and regulating our immune system and mood. The dressing includes miso, a fermented paste made from soya beans, which provides a source of bacteria that may also be supportive for our gut health. This is a meat-free dish but it's pretty 'meaty' for our microbiome.

serves 2

50g red rice (or wild or other rice)

25g pecans, roughly chopped

15g sunflower seeds

75g tenderstem broccoli

75g green beans

2 generous handfuls roughly chopped kale leaves

25g flat-leaf parsley, roughly chopped

½ avocado, sliced

Handful radish sprouts (or alfalfa or other sprouts)

Sea salt

miso mustard dressing

2 tablespoons unpasteurised white miso paste

½ teaspoon yellow mustard powder

1 teaspoon raw honey

3 tablespoons filtered water

Preheat the oven to 150°C/Gas 2.

Cook the rice according to the packet instructions and leave to cool.

Meanwhile, put the chopped pecans and sunflower seeds on a baking tray and roast in the oven for 30 minutes. Remove and leave to cool.

To make the dressing, whisk together the miso paste, mustard and honey until evenly mixed, then whisk in the filtered water.

Steam the broccoli and beans for 5 minutes. Add the kale to the steamer for the final minute.

Add the cooked greens to the cooked rice and combine. Stir through the parsley, dressing and nuts and mix thoroughly. Divide between two shallow bowls. Lay the avocado slices along one side of the bowl, top with the sprouts and sprinkle a pinch of sea salt over each bowl.

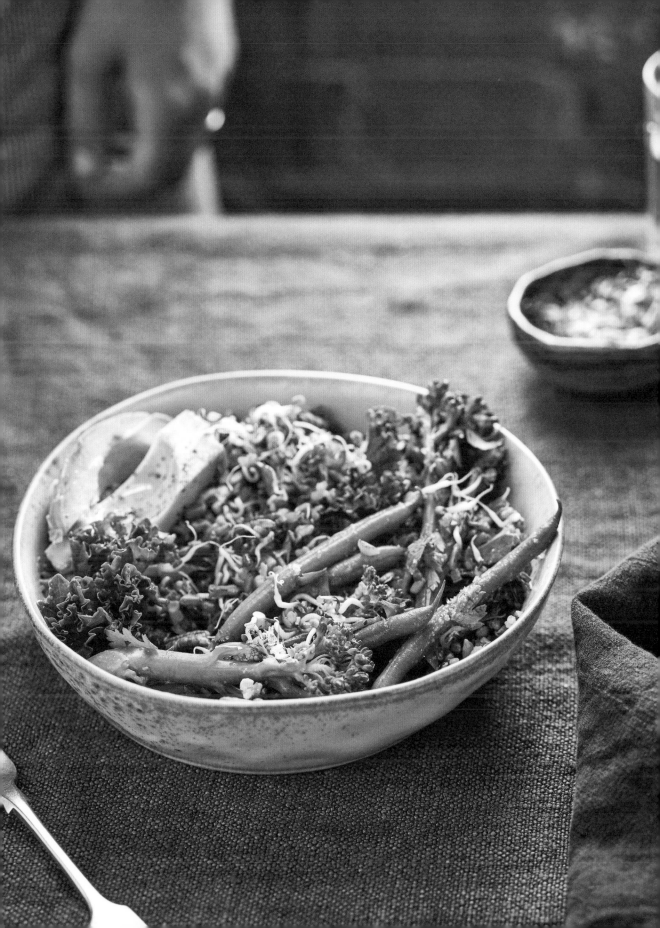

butter bean, roasted red pepper and quinoa salad with chive sour cream

Beans are a super-nutritious food but it's best to soak them to reduce their antinutrient content (see page 65). This recipe is packed with flavour but, for an extra kick, add some finely diced fresh chilli or dried chilli flakes.

serves 2

200g cooked butter beans (see tip)

2 red peppers

50g dried quinoa

2 tablespoons sour cream or crème fraîche (or coconut yogurt for a vegan version)

1 tablespoon finely chopped chives

2 tablespoons chopped fresh parsley

2 tablespoons extra virgin olive oil, plus a little for the peppers

Juice of ½ lemon

Sea salt and black pepper

If cooking the beans from dried, do this first.

Preheat the oven to 200°C/Gas 6. Line a baking tray with baking parchment. Cut the peppers in half lengthways and remove the seeds and stalks. Place on the baking tray, drizzle with a little olive oil and roast for 25–30 minutes until the skins start to blacken. Remove from the oven and leave to cool.

Rinse and drain the quinoa and place in a saucepan with 150ml filtered water. Bring to the boil, cover and simmer for about 10 minutes until all the water has been absorbed and the quinoa is cooked through (you may need to add a bit more water). Once cooked, fluff with a fork and transfer to a large bowl.

In a small bowl, mix together the sour cream and chives.

Slice the peppers into strips and add to the quinoa bowl. Then add the cooked beans, parsley, olive oil, lemon juice and a couple of generous pinches of salt and pepper. Mix thoroughly. Divide between two plates and top with the sour cream.

tip

To cook the amount for this recipe you will need 65g dried butter beans. Soak them overnight in filtered water, drain and rinse. Put them in a large saucepan with 300ml filtered water. Bring slowly to the boil, skim off any froth, then cover and simmer for about 1 hour until tender.

miso slaw

A mouth-watering slaw that combines miso and sauerkraut to provide natural sources of beneficial bacteria to support the gut. This is a great side for sandwiches when you want a substantial lunch and is also the perfect accompaniment to burgers.

serves 3–4

150g sauerkraut, drained

1 carrot, peeled and sliced into matchstick size pieces

½ fennel bulb, very finely sliced

2 tablespoons unpasteurised white miso paste

2 tablespoons mirin or rice wine vinegar

1 tablespoon tamari

1 teaspoon sesame oil

1 tablespoon black sesame seeds

Put the sauerkraut, carrot and fennel in a bowl. Mix evenly – I like to get my hands in here.

In a separate small bowl whisk together the miso paste, mirin, tamari and sesame oil to create a thick dressing.

Add the dressing to the bowl of vegetables, along with the sesame seeds. Mix through evenly – I get my hands in here too. Store in the fridge until ready to serve. This will keep for up to a week.

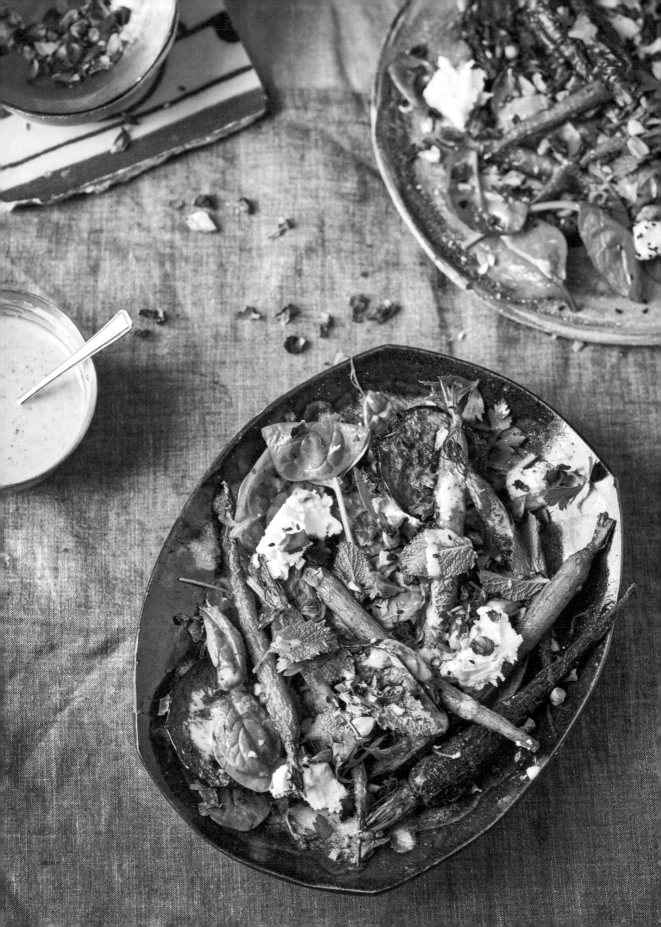

ras el hanout aubergine and carrots, goats' cheese and sumac tahini dressing

This warm melody of colours and flavours is designed to make you and your microbiome smile. As well as being rich in antioxidants and fibre that help your microbiome produce beneficial substances, such as serotonin and butyrate, this recipe includes goats' cheese, a natural source of bacteria believed to be beneficial for our gut. A sprinkling of rose petals gives an extra flourish of love and care to lift your mind too.

serves 2

1 small–medium aubergine (approx. 300g), cut into 5mm slices

150g baby carrots, left whole (or regular carrots, peeled and sliced into batons)

2 teaspoons ras el hanout

1 tablespoon organic butter, melted

100g baby spinach leaves

Handful fresh mint, roughly chopped

Handful fresh parsley, roughly chopped

1 teaspoon nigella seeds

60g unpasteurised soft goats' cheese

1 tablespoon chopped pistachios

Rose petals (optional)

Sea salt

sumac tahini dressing

1 tablespoon tahini

1 tablespoon fresh lemon juice

½ teaspoon sumac

½ teaspoon garlic-infused olive oil

Preheat the oven to 200°C/Gas 6. Line a large baking tray with baking parchment.

Place the aubergine slices and carrots in a large bowl. Add the ras el hanout and melted butter and toss to coat the veg. Spread the aubergines and carrots on the baking tray and roast for 25–30 minutes until nicely browned.

Meanwhile, make the dressing by mixing all the ingredients together in a small bowl.

When the aubergine and carrots are cooked, tip them back into the large bowl and add the spinach, mint and parsley and mix together. Divide between two plates and add the nigella seeds then crumble over the goats' cheese. Drizzle over the tahini dressing and sprinkle with the pistachios and a few rose petals, if using. Finish with a generous pinch of sea salt.

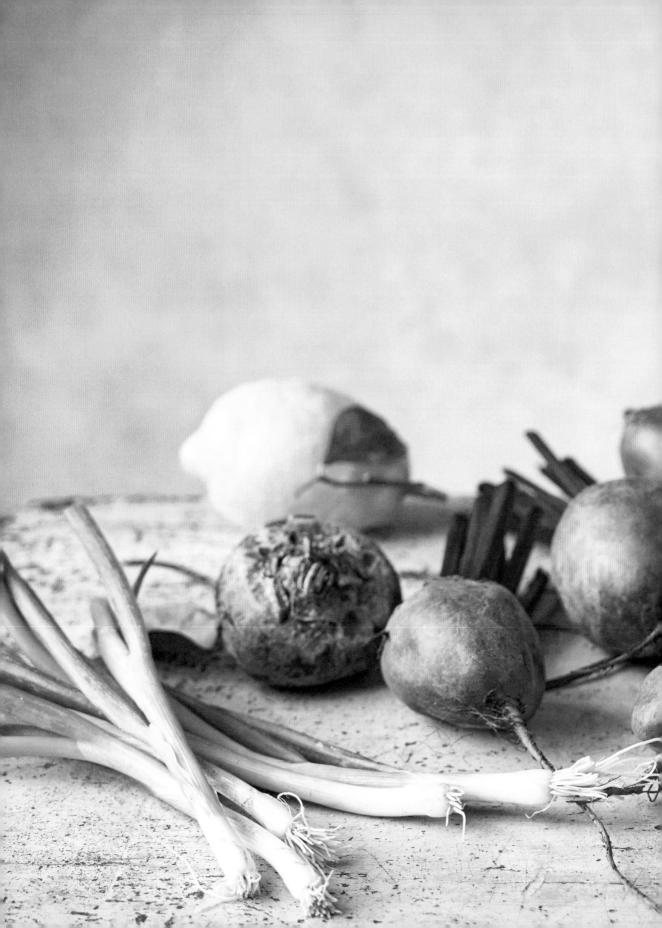

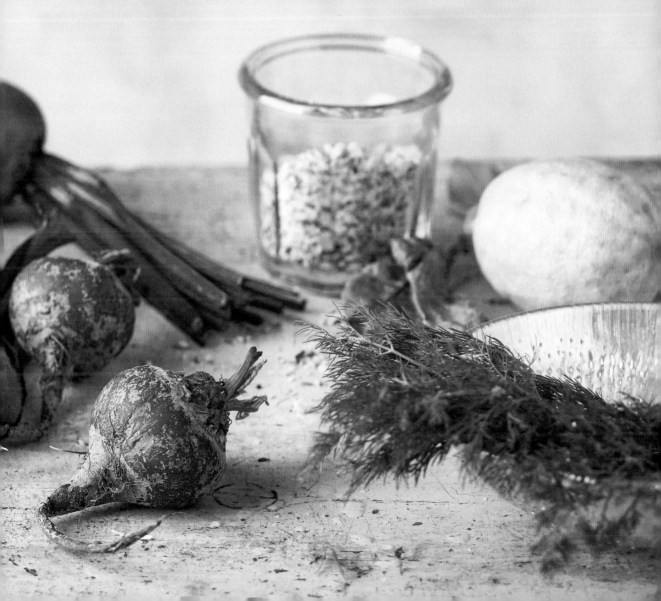

veggie and
vegan mains

smoky tofu with carrot peanut curry

I love this curry, as the subtle smoky flavours combine with the natural sweetness of carrots and a spicy twist to give maximum taste impact. The bold orange and red hues mean that this recipe provides a brilliant melange of antioxidants and fibre that help to support a thriving microbiome.

serves 2

300g non-GMO organic tofu

½ tablespoon arrowroot

2 teaspoons smoked paprika

2 teaspoons ground cumin

½ teaspoon chipotle chilli flakes (or chilli flakes, which won't be as smoky)

1 tablespoon coconut aminos or tamari

Smoked sea salt and black pepper

carrot peanut curry

150g baby carrots

1 tablespoon ghee or organic butter (or coconut oil for a vegan version)

1 garlic clove, crushed

2 teaspoons curry leaves

1 tablespoon mild curry powder

1 tablespoon unsweetened peanut butter (I prefer crunchy but smooth is fine too)

2 tablespoons tomato paste

2 tablespoons fresh lemon juice

100g spinach leaves

1 tablespoon desiccated coconut, plus extra to serve

Fresh coriander to serve

Preheat the oven to 200°C/Gas 6. Line a baking sheet with baking parchment.

To get the tofu crispy you need to remove as much of the excess water as possible, so wrap the tofu in kitchen paper or a light muslin cloth and leave in a colander to drain for 15 minutes. Unwrap and cut into 12 cubes or triangles.

In a large bowl mix the arrowroot, smoked paprika, cumin, chilli flakes and a couple of generous pinches of smoked salt and black pepper. Then add the tofu and coconut aminos and mix to coat the tofu evenly. Place on the baking sheet and bake for 25–30 minutes until golden and crisp.

While the tofu is cooking, make the curry. Steam or lightly boil the carrots until tender then drain. Heat the ghee/butter/coconut oil in a large saucepan over a medium heat. Add the garlic and cook for 1 minute then add the carrots, curry leaves, curry powder, peanut butter, tomato paste and lemon juice, mix together and cook for a further minute. Add the spinach and cook for another minute. Remove from the heat and stir through the coconut.

Serve the curry alongside the tofu and garnish with a sprinkle of coconut and fresh coriander.

Peking jackfruit with sesame rice and hoisin sauce

The texture of jackfruit makes it an excellent meat substitute that is super-satisfying. I've marinated it in some Peking-style spices to give it a hearty flavour, paired it with brown rice to further boost the fibre content of this dish and finished it with a simple hoisin sauce. Tuck in and delight your taste buds and your microbiome.

serves 2

100g brown rice

400g jackfruit chunks (from a jar)

2 teaspoons sesame seeds

⅓ cucumber, sliced into batons

6 spring onions, sliced into batons

jackfruit marinade

1 teaspoon sesame oil

½ teaspoon ground ginger

1 teaspoon Chinese five spice powder

2 tablespoons rice wine vinegar or mirin

1 tablespoon soy sauce (or tamari for a gluten-free version)

hoisin sauce

1 tablespoon soy sauce (or tamari for a gluten-free version)

2 teaspoons rice wine vinegar or mirin

2 tablespoons peanut butter

1 teaspoon maple syrup

¼ teaspoon garlic powder

½ teaspoon sesame oil

Pinch mild chilli powder

3 teaspoons filtered water

To cook the rice, bring 650ml filtered water to the boil in a large saucepan. Add the rice, reduce the heat and simmer for 30 minutes.

Meanwhile, preheat the oven to 200°C/Gas 6. Line a baking tray with baking parchment.

Rinse the jackfruit in a colander, pat dry and place in a large bowl. In a small bowl, whisk together the marinade ingredients then pour over the jackfruit and mix to coat the jackfruit evenly. Place on the baking tray and bake for 20 minutes.

In a small bowl, mix together the hoisin sauce ingredients and place to one side.

Once the rice is cooked, drain off any remaining water and put the rice back into the pan. Add the sesame seeds and cover with a lid. Leave for 10 minutes.

To serve, divide the rice between two shallow bowls. Place the jackfruit on the rice on one side of each bowl. On the other side add the cucumber and spring onion batons and spoon over the hoisin sauce.

tempeh tacos

Great to enjoy with family and friends, this is a really fun, plant-based twist on a taco recipe. It uses fermented soya beans in the form of tempeh and is an easy way to pack in plenty of fibre, antioxidants and bags of flavour that will excite your microbes and your mind – arriba arriba!

serves 3–4

200g romano peppers

1 avocado

Juice of 2 limes

½ tablespoon coconut oil

1 garlic clove, crushed

1 tablespoon smoked paprika

1 tablespoon ground cumin

½ teaspoon chipotle chilli flakes

2 tablespoons coconut aminos

200g non-GMO organic tempeh, sliced into 1cm strips

40g tomato paste

50g cherry tomatoes, halved

12 crispy corn taco shells

Half an iceberg lettuce, shredded

Handful fresh coriander leaves

Sea salt

Lime wedges to serve

Preheat the oven to 200°C/Gas 6. Line a baking tray with baking parchment. Cut the peppers in half lengthways, remove the seeds and stalks and then cut into 2–3cm thick slices. Place on the baking tray and roast for 25–30 minutes.

Meanwhile, cut the avocado in half, remove the stone and scoop out the flesh into a small bowl. Mash the avocado with the lime juice and a couple of generous pinches of sea salt. Place in the fridge until ready to assemble your tacos.

When the peppers are soft, remove from the oven and turn the oven down to 150°C/Gas 2.

In a large frying pan, heat the coconut oil and add the garlic, paprika, cumin, chilli flakes, coconut aminos and tempeh. Cook for 1–2 minutes until the tempeh is coated. Then add the tomato paste, cherry tomatoes and the cooked peppers and cook for a further 1–2 minutes. Take off the heat and put to one side.

Line another baking tray with baking parchment. Lay out your taco shells and place in the oven for 10 minutes.

To assemble the tacos, start with a tablespoon of the mashed avocado, then add a handful of shredded lettuce, 2 tablespoons of the tempeh mix and finish with the coriander leaves. Repeat until you have filled all your taco shells. Serve with lime wedges to squeeze over.

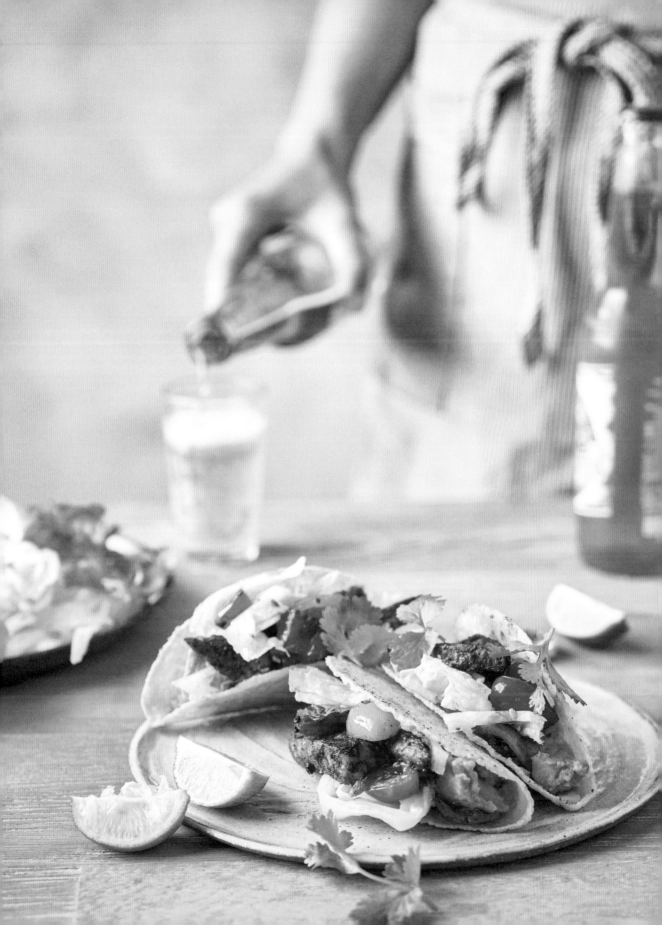

maple-glazed tempeh with broccoli, shiitake and truffle oil

Sticky and sweet, this plant-based dish combines umami flavours, fibre and fermented foods and is finger-licking good for our microbiome as well as our taste buds. Tempeh is made from fermented soya beans and packs in plenty of fibre to support our gut. Shiitake, like other mushrooms, provide an excellent source of prebiotics to feed the microbiome, as do the high amounts of antioxidants in broccoli.

serves 2

200g non-GMO organic tempeh

1 tablespoon maple syrup

1 teaspoon mirin

2 tablespoons tamari

1½ teaspoons sesame oil

50g brown rice

250g tenderstem broccoli

2 tablespoons ghee (or coconut oil for a vegan version)

100g fresh shiitake mushrooms, chopped into 1–2cm pieces

1 teaspoon truffle oil

1 teaspoon black sesame seeds

Cut the block of tempeh into four triangles and place in a shallow dish. Mix together the maple syrup, mirin, 1 tablespoon of the tamari and 1 teaspoon of the sesame oil and pour over the tempeh. Turn it over to coat it in the marinade then cover and leave in the fridge for at least 30 minutes or up to a few hours.

Cook the rice according to the packet instructions. Set aside, cover and keep warm.

Steam the broccoli until tender and set aside.

In a large saucepan, heat half the ghee or oil over a medium heat, reduce the heat and add the tempeh and its marinade. Fry for 5 minutes, turning frequently. Set aside, cover and keep warm.

In a large frying pan, heat the remaining ghee or oil over a medium heat and add the shiitake. Fry for 3–4 minutes and then add the remaining 1 tablespoon of tamari and the cooked broccoli. Cook for a further 1 minute. Remove from the heat.

Add the remaining sesame oil to the brown rice and stir well. Divide the rice between two bowls. Add the broccoli and shiitake and top with the tempeh. Drizzle with the truffle oil and sprinkle over the sesame seeds.

roasted smoky squash, greens and goats' cheese bowl

This dish is like a hug in a bowl on those nights where you feel frazzled and in need of some restorative, nourishing food. You'll be happy to know that your microbes will be similarly restored by the mixture of antioxidants, fibre and fermented foods provided via the squash, cavolo nero and cheese. This has comfort food written all over it.

serves 3–4

2 medium–large squash, such as butternut, acorn, pumpkin

1 tablespoon smoked paprika

1 tablespoon ground cumin

1 tablespoon ground cinnamon

30g organic butter, melted

100g cavolo nero

60g unpasteurised soft goats' cheese

Few sprigs fresh thyme, leaves picked

Sea salt

dressing

2 tablespoons tahini

1 teaspoon garlic-infused olive oil

Generous squeeze lemon juice

2–3 tablespoons filtered water

Preheat the oven to 220°C/Gas 7. Line two baking trays with baking parchment.

Thoroughly wash and/or scrub the squash, keeping the skin on. Cut into wedges and remove the seeds. Place in a large bowl. Add the smoked paprika, cumin and cinnamon and mix to coat the squash evenly. Transfer to the baking trays, drizzle the butter over the squash then roast for 25–30 minutes.

While the squash is cooking, cut the cavolo nero into chunks. Bring a large saucepan of water to the boil, add the cavolo nero then reduce the heat and simmer for 4–5 minutes. Drain in a colander and put to one side.

To make the dressing, mix the tahini, olive oil and lemon juice together to create a paste. Gradually add filtered water to get the consistency you prefer.

Transfer the roasted squash to a big bowl. Add the cooked cavolo nero and mix together. Divide this mixture between individual serving bowls. Top with the goats' cheese, drizzle generously with the tahini dressing and finish with some fresh thyme leaves and a generous pinch of sea salt.

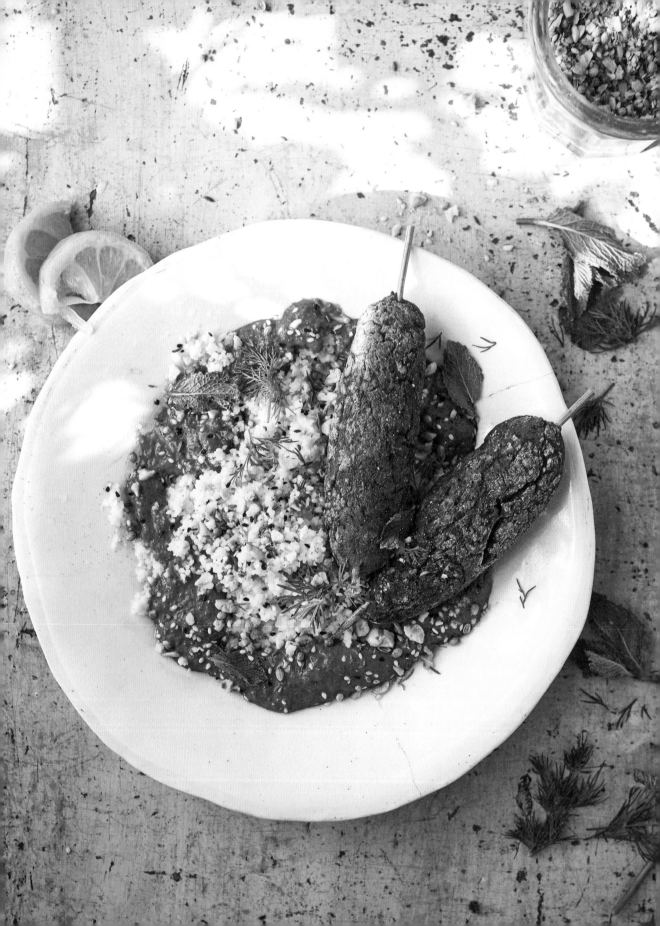

beet kebab couscous bowl with beet borani

Beetroot is the star of this dish and an excellent source of fibre and antioxidants to boost the health of the gut. Chickpeas and chickpea flour are also rich in fibre, to give our microbes something decidedly hearty to chew on.

serves 2

200–250g beetroot, unpeeled

1 tablespoon organic butter (or coconut oil for a vegan version)

2 spring onions, chopped

1 teaspoon dried oregano

2 teaspoons sumac

2 teaspoons ground cumin

1 teaspoon ground coriander

75g cooked chickpeas

100g chickpea flour, plus extra for rolling

20g ground almonds

2 tablespoons roughly chopped fresh parsley

Sea salt and pepper

borani

75g sheep's milk yogurt (or other yogurt of your choice; use coconut yogurt for a vegan version)

1 teaspoon garlic-infused olive oil (or ½ crushed garlic clove and 1 teaspoon extra virgin olive oil)

1 teaspoon tahini

to serve

150g couscous

Squeeze fresh lemon juice

1 tablespoon Dukkah (page 136)

Small handful dill, roughly chopped

10–15 mint leaves, roughly torn

Steam the beetroot for about 60 minutes until cooked through. Leave to cool, then remove the skins by gently rubbing, trim the ends and cut into 3–4cm cubes.

In a large saucepan heat the butter and add the spring onions, half the beetroot, the oregano and spices and fry for 2–3 minutes. Add the chickpeas and cook for a further 2 minutes. Remove from the heat and leave to cool slightly. Put the mixture into a food processor and add the chickpea flour, ground almonds, parsley and a couple of generous pinches of sea salt and pepper. Process until the mixture forms a sticky dough.

Dust a board with chickpea flour, tip the mixture onto the board and roll to coat in the flour. Divide into four balls. Pierce each ball with a skewer and carefully spread the mixture along the skewers to make kebabs around 9–10cm long, pressing the ends firmly. Place in the fridge for at least 20 minutes or up to 4 hours to firm up.

Put the remaining beetroot into a food processor, add the borani ingredients and blend until smooth. Place in the fridge to chill.

Preheat the oven to 180°C/Gas 4 and line a baking tray with baking parchment. Lay the kebabs on the baking tray and bake for 20 minutes, turning halfway through.

Meanwhile, prepare the couscous according to the packet instructions. Squeeze over the lemon juice and add sea salt and pepper to taste. Divide the couscous between two bowls. Spoon the borani around the sides of the bowl then lay the kebabs on top. Sprinkle with the dukkah, dill and mint leaves.

sunshine patties with besan chilla and sweetcorn chilli dip

These patties might take a bit of time, as you have to soak the split peas, but like a lot of things in life they are worth the wait – and the recipe is actually really simple. Yellow split peas are an excellent source of fibre and plant-based protein. Traditional Indian chickpea flour pancakes and a sweetcorn dip really up the ante with legumes that provide a wealth of fibre to keep our microbiome sprightly.

serves 2

sunshine patties

100g yellow split peas

50g carrots

2 tablespoons roughly chopped fresh parsley

25g chickpea flour

1 tablespoon sesame seeds

1 tablespoon fresh lemon juice

¼ teaspoon garlic powder

1 teaspoon onion powder

1 teaspoon ground galangal (or ½ teaspoon ground ginger)

1 teaspoon ground coriander

1 teaspoon ground cumin

1 teaspoon ground turmeric

Generous pinch of sea salt and black pepper

besan chilla

75g chickpea flour

½ teaspoon bicarbonate of soda

1 tablespoon apple cider vinegar

100ml filtered water

Ghee or organic butter for frying (or coconut oil for a vegan version)

sweetcorn chilli dip

200g cooked sweetcorn

1 teaspoon cumin

2 tablespoons grated Parmesan (or nutritional yeast flakes for a vegan version)

1 teaspoon garlic-infused olive oil

Pinch chipotle chilli flakes (or other chilli flakes)

¼–½ teaspoon harissa paste (optional)

Soak the split peas for 5 hours. Drain and rinse. Bring a pan of water to the boil, add the split peas and simmer for 15 minutes. Drain and leave to cool.

Preheat the oven to 200°C/Gas 6. Line a baking tray with baking parchment. Add all the pattie ingredients – except the split peas – to a food processor and pulse until the carrot is finely shredded. Add the split peas and process to form a dough. Transfer to a bowl and add more chickpea flour if it's a bit sticky. Divide the dough into four patties, around 2cm thick. Place on the baking tray and bake for 20 minutes, turning halfway through.

While they are cooking, make the sweetcorn dip. Place all the ingredients in a food processor with a couple of generous pinches of sea salt and blend to a thick dip consistency. Transfer to a bowl.

To make the besan chilla, put the chickpea flour in a bowl, add the bicarbonate of soda, vinegar, water and a pinch of sea salt and whisk all the ingredients together. Let sit for 5 minutes. Heat a frying pan over a medium heat. Add 2 tablespoons of ghee, butter or coconut oil and when hot, add tablespoons of the chickpea batter, spacing them well apart; cook for 4–5 minutes on one side, then flip and cook for another 2 minutes. You should be able to make about eight pancakes, in two batches; add a little more ghee if necessary.

Remove the patties from the oven and serve with the besan chilla, a couple of tablespoons of the sweetcorn dip and a green salad.

dukkah cauliflower 'steak' with green tahini, spinach, curd and capers

You could say that this is as 'meaty' as it gets for your microbiome, due to the feast of fibre the cauliflower provides. The curd or cheese is a natural fermented source of bacteria that is beneficial for our gut health, and a punchy green dressing delights the eyes as well as the taste buds.

serves 2

1 medium–large cauliflower
1–2 tablespoons organic butter
1 tablespoon Dukkah (page 136)
200g baby spinach leaves
100g ewe's curd (or unpasteurised soft goats' cheese)
2 teaspoons capers
1 teaspoon nigella seeds
Sea salt

green tahini

1 tablespoon tahini
1 tablespoon finely chopped fresh parsley
1 tablespoon olive oil
Juice of ½ lemon

Preheat the oven to 200°C/Gas 6. Line a baking tray with baking parchment.

Cut the cauliflower vertically into 'steaks' about 2–3cm thick – you should get around four steaks from the cauliflower. Lay them on the baking tray.

In a saucepan, melt the butter and drizzle over the cauliflower. Put the pan to one side as you will use it for the spinach. Divide the dukkah evenly over the cauliflower steaks, then bake for 30 minutes.

Meanwhile, make the green tahini dressing. In a small bowl mix the tahini, parsley, olive oil and lemon juice. Set aside.

About 5 minutes before the cauliflower is due out of the oven, add the spinach to the saucepan and cook over a medium heat until it has wilted. Divide between two plates.

Place two cauliflower steaks on each plate. Crumble the curd over the steaks and add the capers. Drizzle with a generous tablespoon of the tahini dressing, sprinkle over the nigella seeds and season with sea salt.

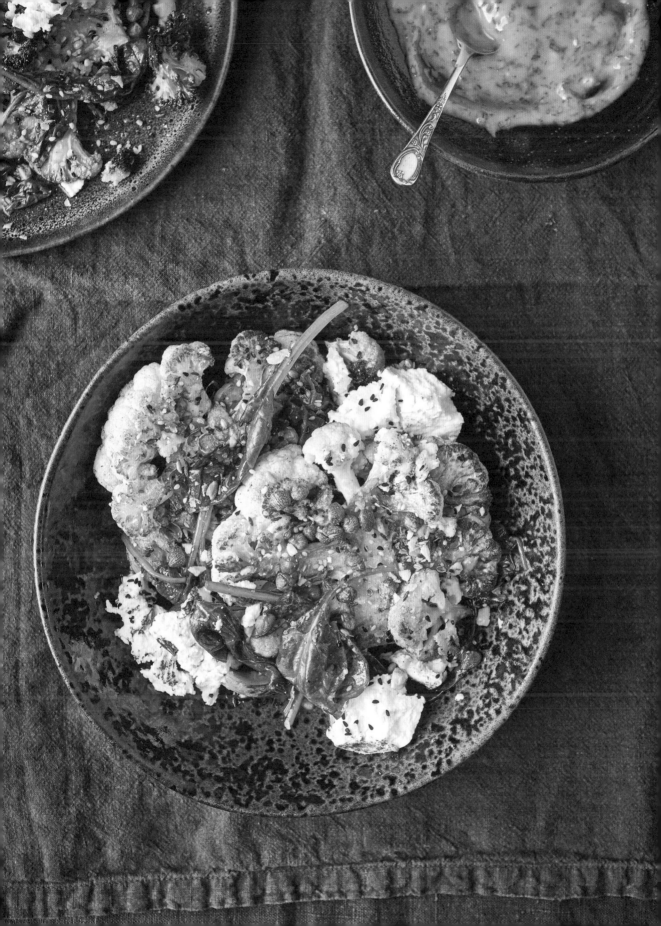

dukkah

Once you start making your own dukkah you won't look back. You'll be chucking it on anything and everything, from scrambled eggs to salads, using it to season fish such as salmon or even scattering it over porridge. Great for your gut and brain as the spicy seeds are plentiful in antioxidants and polyphenols that help to support them both.

makes 1 small jar

75g chopped roasted hazelnuts

2 tablespoons sunflower seeds, crushed

2 tablespoons coriander seeds

2 tablespoons sesame seeds

1 tablespoon cumin seeds

1 teaspoon fennel seeds

1 teaspoon nigella seeds

½ teaspoon sea salt

Pinch black pepper

Preheat the oven to 150°C/Gas 2. Line a baking tray with baking parchment.

Mix all the ingredients together, place on the baking tray and bake for 15 minutes.

Remove from the oven and leave to cool completely before storing in an airtight jar. It will keep for about 1 month.

tips

You can buy ready roasted and chopped hazelnuts, or buy them blanched and roast them in the oven at 150°C/Gas 2 for 20 minutes until golden brown, then chop into small pieces.

Once you know you like dukkah you may want to double up all the ingredients to fill a large jar.

asparagus, feta and pea fritatta

For me, this frittata speaks of springtime, since that is when asparagus is in season in the UK. Choosing ingredients that are local and seasonal is important for many reasons: better nutritionally, better for the planet, and usually a better flavour. And when food tastes better we tend to be more focused while eating it. Asparagus is also an excellent prebiotic to support gut and brain health. This dish keeps well in the fridge, so if making for one you can enjoy it again the next day.

serves 2

240g asparagus
4 large organic eggs
1 tablespoon organic butter
75g frozen peas
75g feta
Handful fresh basil leaves
Sea salt and black pepper

Preheat the oven to 180°C/Gas 4.

Slice off the asparagus tips and put to one side. Trim the woody ends and then quarter the lower part of the asparagus lengthways into fine slices.

Whisk the eggs in a bowl and season well.

Heat a frying pan with an ovenproof handle over a medium heat. Add the butter and, when melted, add the peas and sliced asparagus and cook for 5 minutes, stirring occasionally.

Make sure the asparagus and peas are spread evenly across the pan then carefully pour in the eggs and place the asparagus tips evenly over the eggs. Crumble over the feta and add the basil leaves. Cook until starting to firm around the edges and then place in the oven for 10 minutes.

Carefully remove the pan from the oven, using an oven glove or a tea towel around the handle. Transfer to a large plate. Slice into four and serve two slices per person, with a green salad on the side.

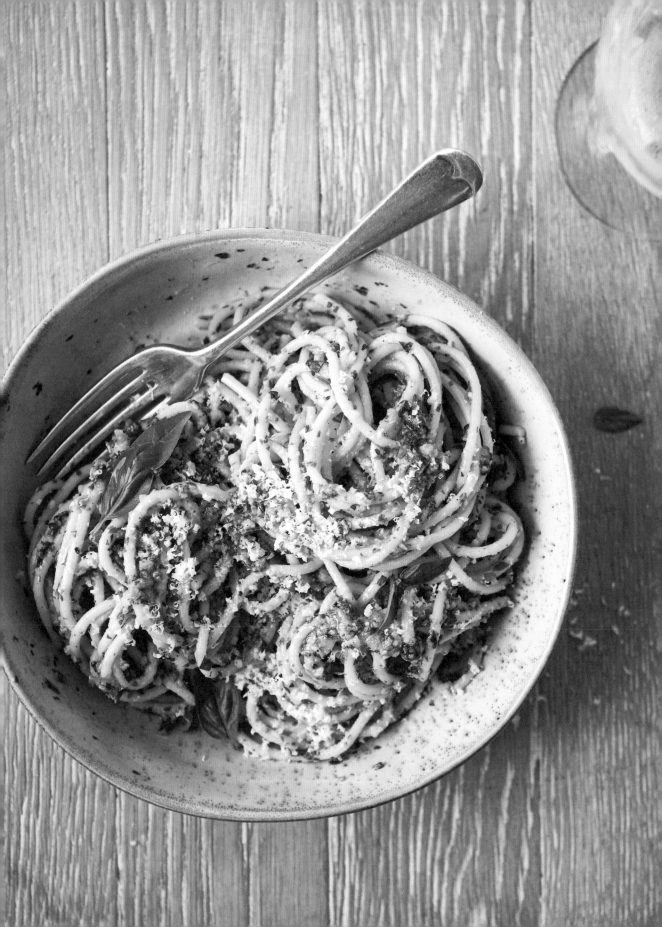

spaghetti with wild garlic pesto

Whenever I feel like making something that is going to bring me comfort and joy, spaghetti is right up there. Here I've combined it with a simple fresh pesto recipe, ideally made from wild garlic, which has an incredible flavour. Garlic is one of the more potent prebiotics that help to stimulate the growth of our microbiome, but if wild garlic is not in season you can use rocket or watercress.

serves 2

50g pine nuts
50g wild garlic leaves (when out of season, replace with rocket or watercress and a fresh garlic clove)
Small handful fresh parsley
50g Parmesan, grated, plus extra to serve (see tip)
Squeeze fresh lemon juice
Sea salt and black pepper
100ml extra virgin olive oil
150g spaghetti

Place the pine nuts on a baking tray and roast at 150°C/Gas 2 for about 20 minutes until golden brown. Set aside to cool. If you want to save time, you can toast them in a dry pan over a gentle heat, but oven-roasting gives a richer flavour.

Put the pine nuts in a food processor and add the wild garlic, parsley, Parmesan, lemon juice and a pinch of sea salt and black pepper. Pulse to break down the ingredients for a minute or so and then gradually add the olive oil until evenly blended. Transfer to a sealable glass or ceramic container and store in the fridge. This will keep for up to 1 week.

Cook the spaghetti until al dente. Drain and then stir through 2 generous tablespoons of the pesto and top with a little – or a lot – more Parmesan.

tips

Gluten-free alternatives to pasta are readily available, so there is no need to miss out if you gut is gluten-sensitive.

Parmesan is an unpasteurised cheese made using animal rennet: vegetarian versions of Italian hard cheese can be substituted.

wine pairing

A simple pasta dish like this matches well with a Verdicchio or unoaked Chardonnay. Or if red is your thing then go for a Teroldego or a young Australian Shiraz.

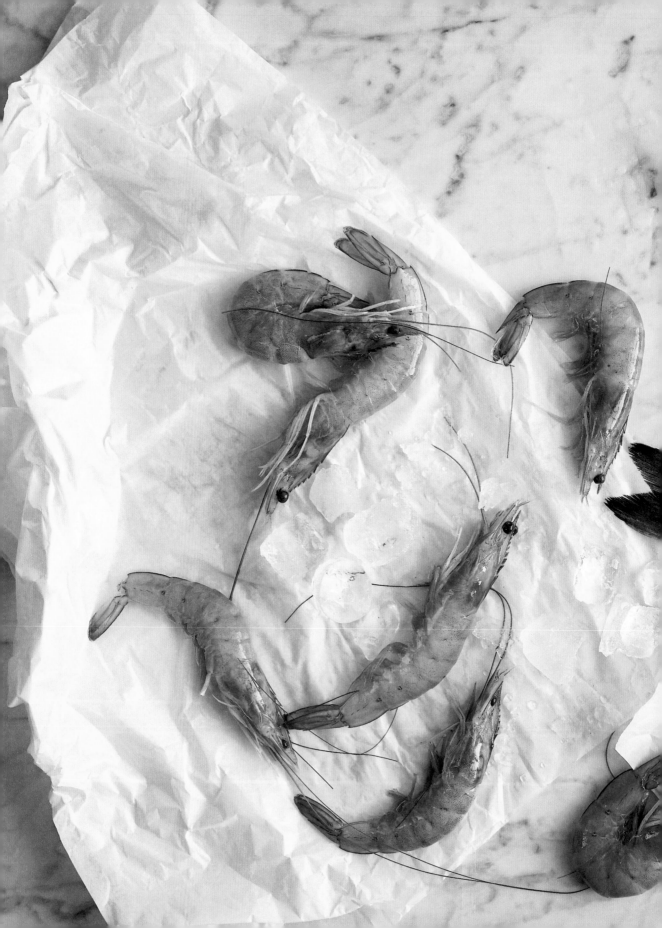

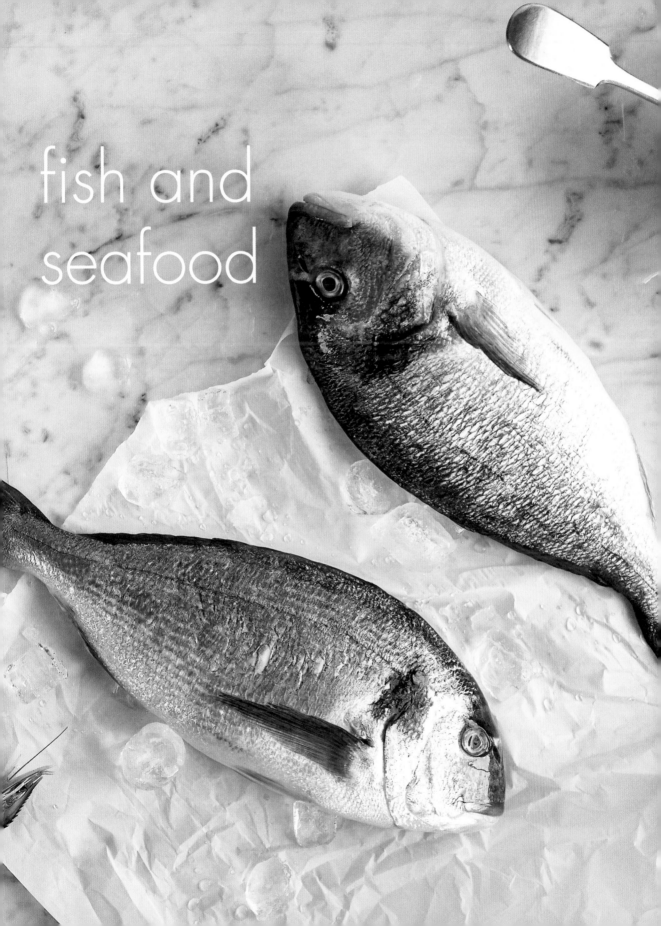

fish and
seafood

smoked mackerel with caponata and lemon yogurt dressing

I think caponata is one of the most glorious things to eat and it features a colourful array of vegetables that make it very attractive for your gut and brain. Omega 3-rich mackerel is the perfect flavour partner, providing essential fatty acids for your microbiome and grey matter. A glass of crisp white wine on the side wouldn't go amiss.

serves 2

2 cooked smoked mackerel fillets

caponata

20g organic butter

1 red onion, thinly sliced

1 aubergine, cut into 3cm cubes

1 celery stalk, cut into 1cm slices

200g cherry or plum tomatoes, halved

2 tablespoons tomato paste

35g pitted green olives, sliced in half or quarters, depending on size – I love big green Cerignola Sicilian ones

2 tablespoons capers

1 tablespoon balsamic vinegar

50ml filtered water

1 teaspoon extra virgin olive oil

1 tablespoon pine nuts, toasted

Small handful fresh basil leaves

Sea salt and black pepper

lemon yogurt dressing

3 tablespoons full fat natural yogurt

1 tablespoon fresh lemon juice

1 teaspoon extra virgin olive oil

¼ teaspoon mustard powder

First make the caponata. Heat the butter in a saucepan over a medium–high heat. Add the onion and fry for 3 minutes. Then add the aubergine and celery and cook for 7 minutes. Turn the heat down to low. Add the tomatoes, tomato paste, olives, capers and vinegar and season with a pinch of sea salt and black pepper. Then add the water and stir well. Cover and simmer for 10 minutes.

Meanwhile, mix together the ingredients for the yogurt dressing and place in the fridge.

Remove the caponata from the heat and leave to cool to room temperature. Add the olive oil and toasted pine nuts. Mix through and top with the basil leaves.

Serve the mackerel with as much of the caponata as you like and then dot over the yogurt dressing.

tip

You can store the caponata in the fridge for up to 3 days. Pair leftover caponata with scrambled eggs on sourdough toast for a beautiful Sicilian-inspired brunch.

spicy wild salmon with celeriac saag aloo

I first discovered amchoor around 15 years ago and to my delight it is now widely available. An Indian spice made from green unripe mangoes, amchoor has a distinct citrusy yet spicy flavour. Combined with turmeric and cumin it gives a beautiful golden colour and rich flavour to the salmon. Turmeric is a spice that has been used extensively as a medicinal herb in India for hundreds of years and has been heralded for its brain-supportive attributes due to the compound curcumin, although (as current science tells us) you do have to eat rather a lot to get the benefits. I've swapped the traditional potatoes of sag aloo for celeriac, as I like the flavour in this particular dish, but you can always use spuds instead if you prefer.

serves 2

1 tablespoon amchoor

2 teaspoons ground cumin

4 teaspoons ground turmeric

2 wild salmon fillets

1 small–medium celeriac (about 450g), peeled and chopped into 5cm cubes

10g organic butter

1 small onion, finely sliced

½ red chilli, finely diced

1 garlic clove, crushed

200g fresh spinach leaves

Sea salt

Mix the amchoor, cumin and half the turmeric together and rub over the salmon fillets. Leave for 20–30 minutes.

Steam or lightly boil the celeriac until just tender, then drain and put to one side.

Preheat the grill to medium. Cook the salmon under the grill for about 5–10 minutes until cooked through (timing will depend on the thickness of the fillets).

Melt the butter in a large saucepan over a medium heat, add the onion, chilli and garlic and cook for about 5 minutes until the onion has softened slightly. Then add the cooked celeriac, spinach and the remaining 2 teaspoons of turmeric and cook until the spinach has wilted down.

Divide the spinach mix between two plates and top with the cooked salmon. Season with a pinch of sea salt.

wild salmon, pak choi and leeks with sesame ponzu sauce

Fuss-free and flavoursome, this recipe features wild salmon as the headline act, although arguably it's the sesame ponzu that really elevates the dish. Boasting omega-3s that are important for brain health and mood, as well as supporting our microbiome, this dish will help to spark an inner sense of positivity.

serves 2

2 wild salmon fillets

3 tablespoons coconut aminos

1 tablespoon sesame seeds

2 leeks

200g pak choi

½ teaspoon sesame oil

2 teaspoons yuzu juice (or a mix of fresh lemon juice and orange juice)

Sea salt

Preheat the oven to 180°C/Gas 4. Line a baking tray with baking parchment.

Place the salmon on the baking tray. Drizzle 1 tablespoon of the coconut aminos over the fillets, sprinkle with half the sesame seeds and season generously with sea salt. Bake for 20–25 minutes.

Meanwhile, prepare the leeks and pak choi. Slice the leeks on a slight diagonal angle to around 2cm thick. Separate the leaves of the pak choi and trim off the thicker ends of the stems. Bring a large saucepan of water to the boil. Around 5–10 minutes before the salmon is due to finish cooking, add the leeks to the boiling water; after around 3–4 minutes add the pak choi and boil for a further minute. Drain and place on kitchen paper to absorb excess water.

Remove the salmon from the oven and leave to sit for a couple of minutes while you make the ponzu sauce. In a small bowl, mix the remaining 2 tablespoons of coconut aminos and ½ tablespoon of sesame seeds with the sesame oil and yuzu juice.

To serve, divide the leeks and pak choi between two plates, add the salmon and drizzle the ponzu sauce over the dish. Finish with a pinch of sea salt.

wine pairing

Try an Albariño, Sancerre or unoaked Chenin Blanc; if you prefer red, try a Gamay (such as Beaujolais) or a young Pinot Noir.

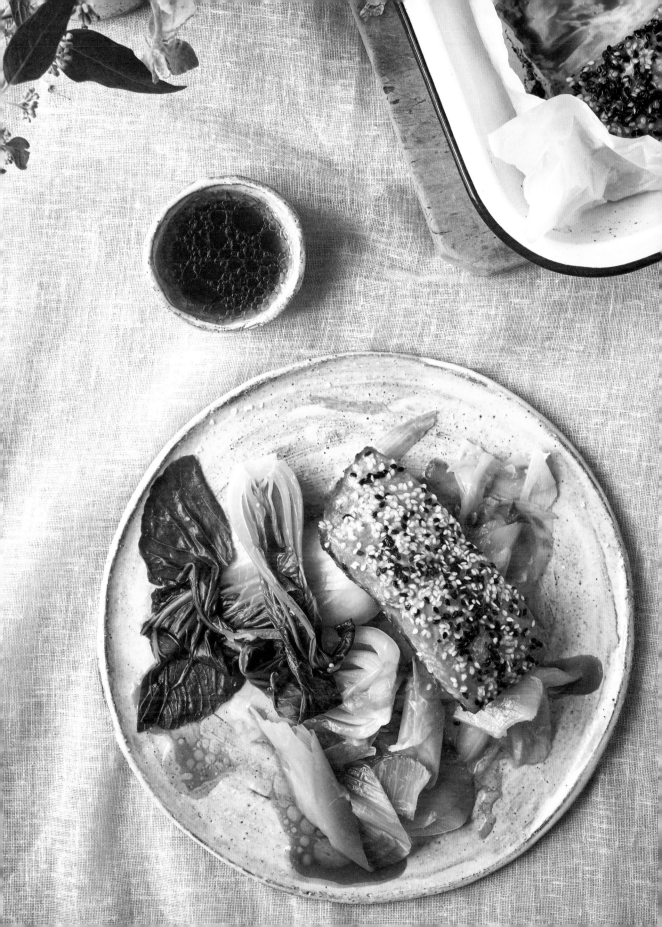

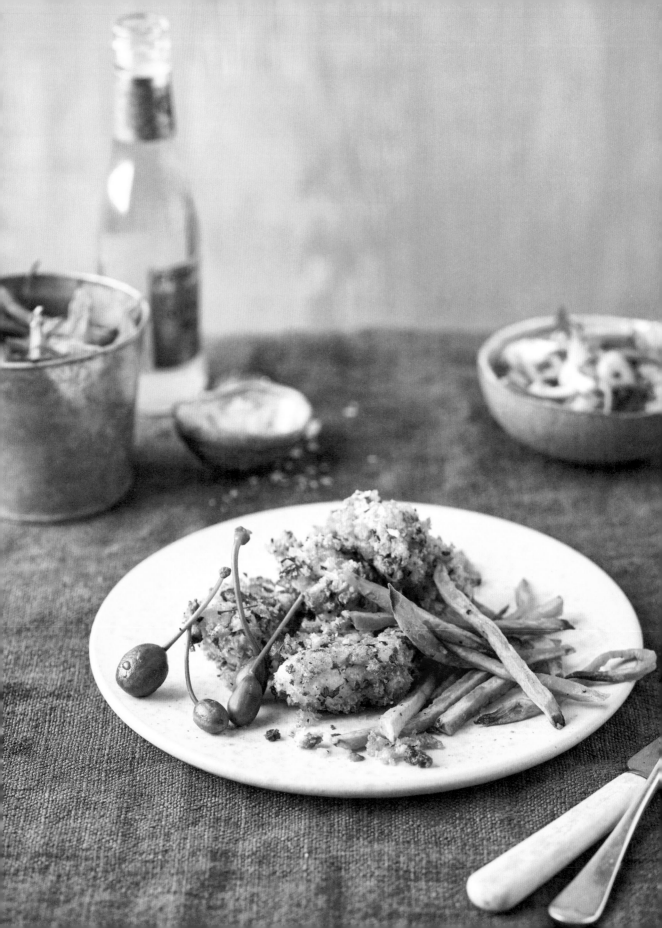

monkfish nuggets with sweet potato fries

Fish and chips with a twist. I've coated the nuggets in sourdough breadcrumbs as they can be easier for some people to digest than regular breadcrumbs. That's likely to be due to the fermentation process by which sourdough is made, which means it's almost 'pre-digested' for us. The sweet potatoes provide a generous amount of beta-carotene, an antioxidant that helps to support the health of the microbiome and brain. A side of Miso Slaw (page 119) goes well with this.

serves 2

2 slices fresh sourdough bread

300g monkfish fillet, cut into 5cm pieces

30g coconut flour

1 organic egg

½ tablespoon finely chopped fresh parsley

Grated zest of ½ lemon

½ tablespoon extra virgin olive oil

Sea salt and black pepper

Caperberries or gherkins to serve

sweet potato fries

300g sweet potatoes

1 tablespoon organic butter, melted

Preheat the oven to 180°C/Gas 4.

Put the sourdough in the oven for 10 minutes until it is dry. Break it up and blitz in a food processor to make fine breadcrumbs.

To make the sweet potato fries: line a baking tray with baking parchment. Peel the sweet potatoes and cut into 5mm thick fries. Place in a large bowl and pour over the melted butter; toss to coat evenly and season well with sea salt and pepper. Spread evenly on the baking tray and cook for 20 minutes.

Pat the fish dry with kitchen paper. Now set up the stations for your fish crumbing. Put the coconut flour with a pinch of sea salt and pepper on a tray or a sheet of baking paper. Whisk the egg in a bowl. In a large bowl combine the sourdough breadcrumbs, parsley, lemon zest and olive oil and mix well. Line a baking tray with baking parchment for the finished nuggets.

Taking one piece of fish at a time, coat it in the coconut flour, then dip it into the egg and finally coat it in the breadcrumbs. Place on the lined baking tray.

When you have coated all the fish, place the baking tray in the oven. At this point you can flip your fries. Bake the nuggets and the fries for a further 30 minutes.

To serve, add a final flourish of sea salt to the fries and serve with caperberries or gherkins, and a side of Miso Slaw (page 119) if you like.

rainbow trout miso soba bowl

This dish combines a plethora of flavours. The miso paste gives a distinct umami, sour and salty flavour that sits well alongside the slight bitterness of the greens. Mirin provides sweetness and the trout has abundant omega 3 fatty acids for a healthy microbiome and mind. With a kick of chilli and warming garlic this is a flavour sensation in a bowl.

serves 2

1 tablespoon unpasteurised white miso paste

1 tablespoon mirin

2 wild rainbow trout fillets

100g buckwheat soba noodles

½ tablespoon coconut oil

100g green beans

200g asparagus, trimmed

Handful of spinach leaves

½ red chilli, finely sliced

2 garlic cloves, crushed

Sesame oil to drizzle

Sesame seeds to garnish

In a large shallow dish, mix together the miso paste and mirin. Add the fish and turn it to coat it with the mixture. Place in the fridge for at least 30 minutes.

Preheat the oven to 200°C/Gas 6. Line a baking tray with foil, put the fillets on the tray and bake for 20 minutes until the fish is cooked through.

Meanwhile, bring a large saucepan of water to the boil. Add the soba noodles and make sure they are fully submerged. Let the water return to the boil, then reduce the heat and simmer the noodles according to the packet instructions (usually around 5 minutes but don't overcook them).

While the noodles are cooking, get your colander ready and fill a large bowl with cold water – throw in a couple of ice cubes if you like. Once the noodles are cooked, drain them in the colander and then tip them into the bowl of cold water. Give them a good wash, rubbing well to remove the starch as that's what makes them gummy. Drain again in the colander and let them sit while you cook your veggies.

In a large frying pan or wok, heat the coconut oil and add the green beans and asparagus. Add a splash of water to help them steam. Cook for 3–4 minutes and then add the spinach, chilli and garlic. Cook for a further 1–2 minutes.

Divide the noodles between two bowls, then add the greens and top with the fish. Drizzle with sesame oil and add a generous sprinkling of sesame seeds.

crispy prawns with chilli fennel and smoky paprika dip

Crispy chilli prawns, the beautiful anise flavours of fennel and an undertone of warming spice makes for a really satisfying supper that's quick to prepare. Fennel is renowned for its soothing digestive properties so it's a good choice to restore some calm to the gut and in turn leave the mind feeling more serene too.

serves 2

200g peeled large/jumbo tiger prawns

2 teaspoons arrowroot

½ teaspoon chipotle chilli flakes

2 tablespoons coconut flour

1 organic egg

Sea salt

chilli fennel

1 tablespoon organic butter

2 fennel bulbs, trimmed and thinly sliced

1 teaspoon finely sliced red chilli

1 garlic clove, crushed

Extra virgin olive oil to drizzle

smoky paprika dip

2 tablespoons good quality mayonnaise

Juice of 1 lime

1 teaspoon smoked paprika

Preheat the oven to 200°C/Gas 6. Line a baking tray with baking parchment.

To prepare the prawns, combine the arrowroot, chilli flakes, coconut flour and a pinch of sea salt in a bowl and mix well. Gently pat the prawns on kitchen paper to remove excess moisture. Whisk the egg in a small bowl. Dip the prawns in the egg and then into the arrowroot mix, toss to coat evenly and then place on the baking tray. Pop into the oven and bake for 30 minutes, turning halfway through.

To make the dip, combine the mayo with the lime juice, paprika and a pinch of sea salt. Place in the fridge.

For the chilli fennel, heat the butter in a large frying pan. Add the fennel and fry for about 5 minutes until the fennel begins to brown. Then add the chilli and garlic and fry for a further 2 minutes.

Divide the fennel between two plates and drizzle with the olive oil. Place the prawns on the side. Add a generous tablespoon of the dip, or serve it in a small dipping bowl if you prefer – I like it that way!

baked bream, fennel and tomatoes

This simple baked dish combines beautiful bream with the soothing properties of fennel. It's a sublime combination that is bound to make you feel altogether more present with what is on your plate. Serve with crusty fresh sourdough and a bowl of olive oil and balsamic for dipping. Mediterranean done simply and deliciously!

serves 2

2 fennel bulbs, trimmed and cut into 1cm thick slices
Extra virgin olive oil to drizzle
125g cherry tomatoes
2 sea bream fillets, scaled
6 thin slices lemon
Sea salt
Handful dill fronds
Handful fresh tarragon leaves

Preheat the oven to 200°C/Gas 6. Line a baking tray with foil.

Lay the fennel on the baking tray and drizzle with olive oil. Bake for 15 minutes.

Scatter the tomatoes over the fennel and lay the bream fillets on top, skin side down. Arrange the lemon slices on the fish, add a generous drizzle of olive oil and season with a generous pinch of sea salt. Bake for a further 25 minutes.

Remove from the oven, scatter over the herbs and serve.

wine pairing

This dish goes well with a Sauvignon Blanc or young unoaked Chardonnay.

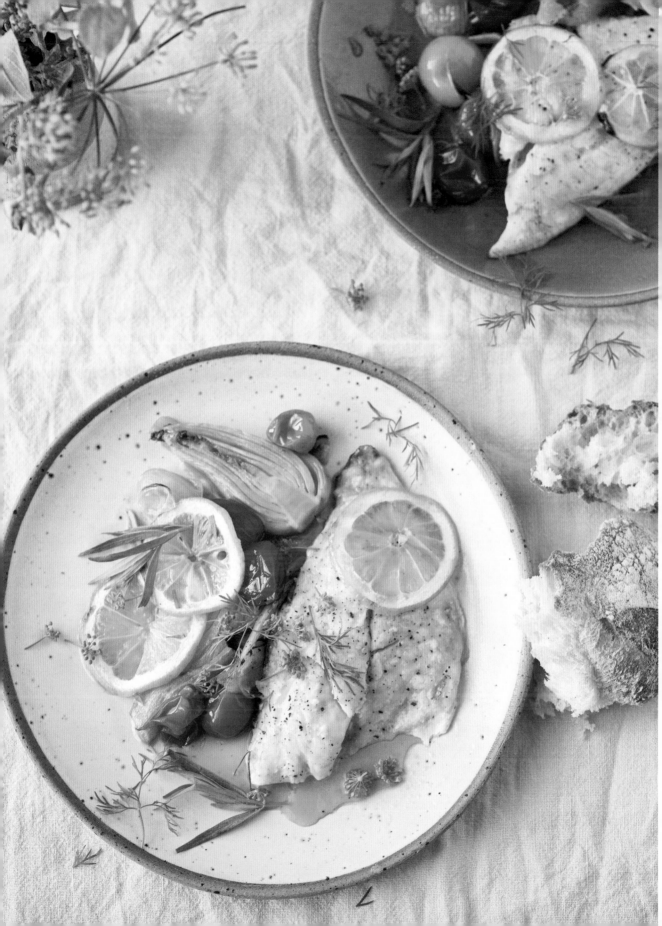

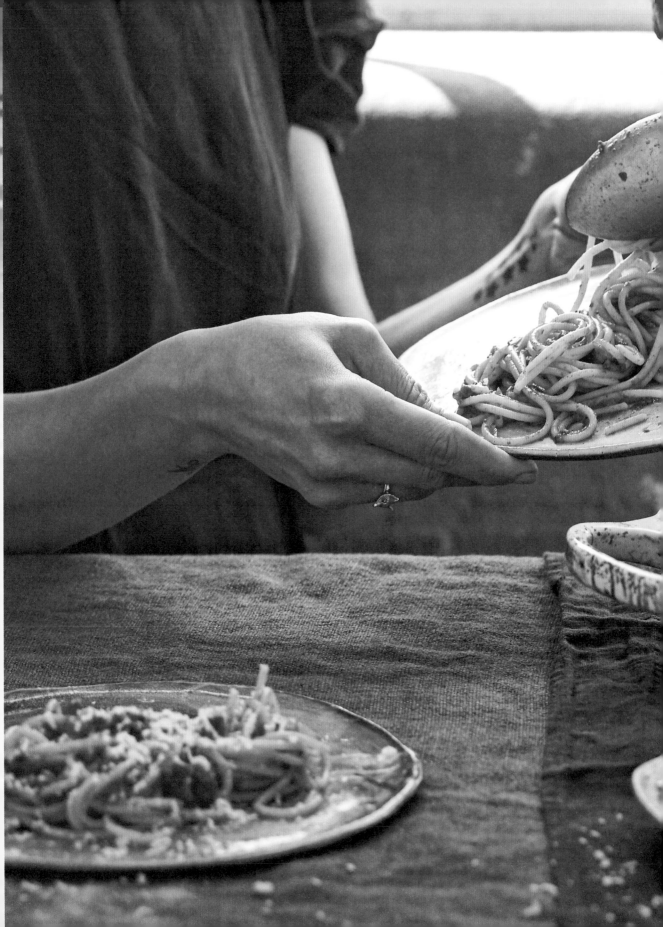

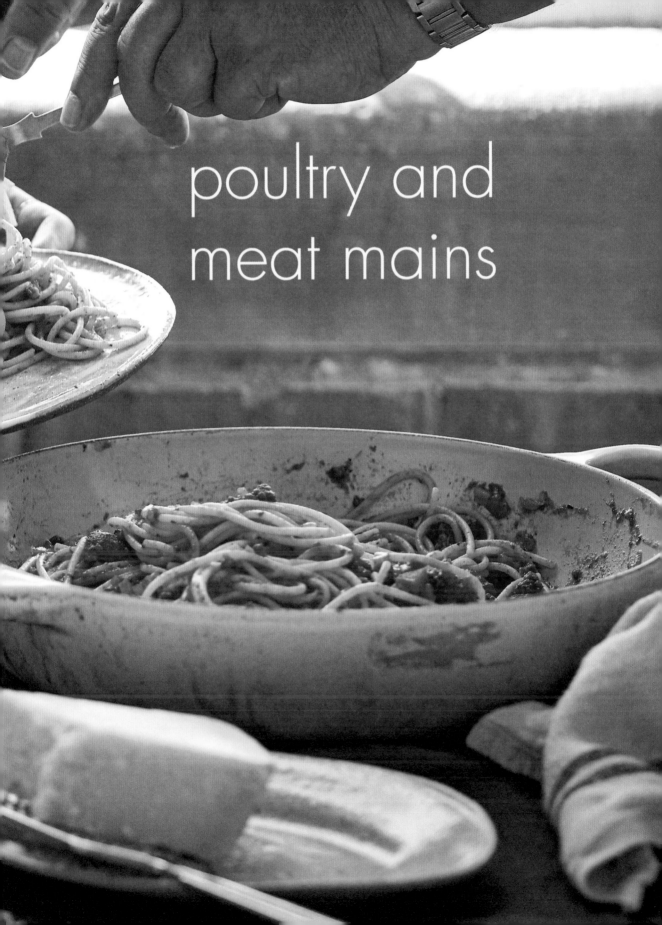

poultry and
meat mains

duck breast, leeks with fennel seeds and spicy carrot purée

Duck is a good source of monounsaturated fat (the type found in olive oil) and healthy saturated fats that have positive benefits for our brain. I've paired it with prebiotic leeks, digestive-soothing fennel seeds and a spicy carrot purée to provide a feast of fibre for your microbiome.

serves 2

2 free range duck breasts
2 leeks, finely sliced
1 tablespoon organic butter
1 teaspoon fennel seeds
Sea salt and black pepper

spicy carrot purée

300g carrots, roughly chopped
2 tablespoons extra virgin olive oil
1 tablespoon organic butter or ghee
2 teaspoons ground cumin
1 teaspoon ground turmeric
1 teaspoon ground cinnamon
1 teaspoon onion powder
½ teaspoon ground fenugreek
¼ teaspoon garlic powder

Preheat the oven to 200°C/Gas 6.

First steam or boil the carrots until tender.

Meanwhile, score the skin of the duck breasts in diagonal lines. Season with salt and pepper. Place the duck breasts skin side down in a cold non-stick frying pan. Place the pan over a medium heat and cook for 5–7 minutes until the skin is golden brown. Using tongs, turn the breasts over and seal on the other side for about a minute. Transfer the breasts, skin side up, to a rack in a roasting pan and roast for 15 minutes.

When the carrots are cooked, drain and place in a blender with the remaining purée ingredients and a pinch of salt and pepper and blend until smooth.

Remove the duck from the oven and leave to rest for 5–10 minutes.

Pan-fry the leeks in the butter, adding a splash of water to help them steam, for 3–4 minutes. Add the fennel seeds and cook for a further minute.

Divide the carrot purée between two plates and serve the leeks alongside. Slice the duck breasts on the diagonal and lay on top of the carrot purée.

wine pairing

If you haven't tried orange wines this might your moment to give them a go, as they can be a great companion to this dish. Their orange colour is due to the fact that they are made from white grapes fermented in their skins. Look for examples from Italy, Slovenia and Georgia.

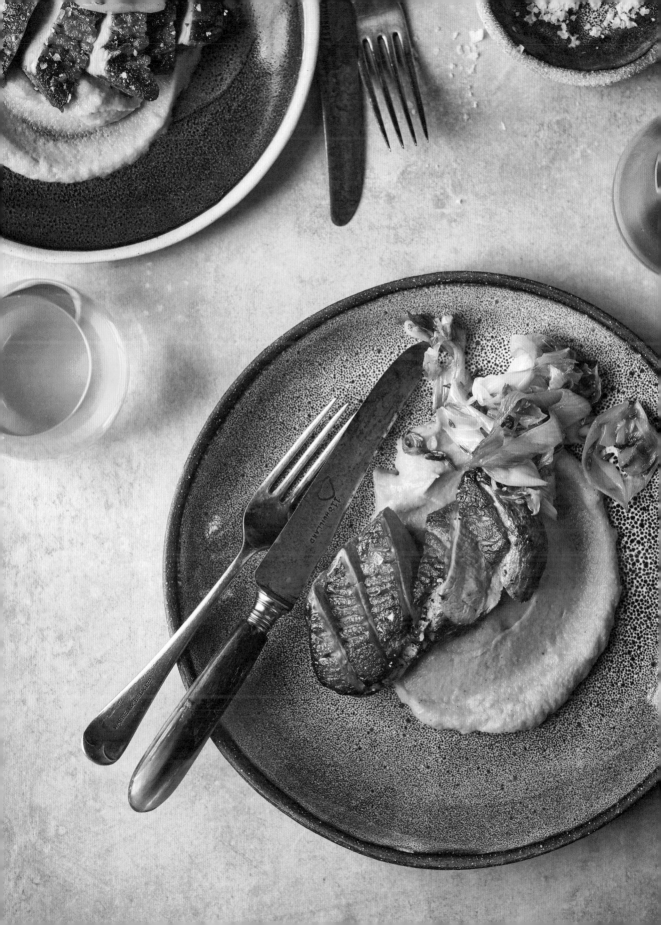

jungle curry

The medley of vegetables in this colourful curry provides different kinds of fibre and a diverse range of antioxidants to help to spice up the microbiome mix. Curries are ace for family suppers and this one can be cooked and on the table in less than 20 minutes. It also freezes well if you want to divide between meals.

serves 4

2 tablespoons ghee or organic butter

2 organic free range chicken breasts, cut into small chunks

150g green beans, trimmed and halved

125g baby sweetcorn

100g sugar snap peas

325ml organic chicken bone broth

4–5 dried lime leaves

2 teaspoons arrowroot whisked with a little water to make a thick paste

50g baby spinach leaves

Small handful fresh basil leaves

Basmati or other rice to serve

curry paste

1 lemongrass stalk

2 teaspoons ground galangal (or ½ teaspoon ground ginger)

2 tablespoons coconut aminos

½ teaspoon mild chilli powder

2 teaspoons ground coriander

2 teaspoons ground cumin

1 garlic clove, crushed

Juice of 1 lime

Sea salt

First make the curry paste. Remove the outer layers of the lemongrass stalk then very finely slice the stalk on the diagonal. Put the sliced lemongrass in a small bowl and add the galangal (or ginger), coconut aminos, chilli powder, coriander, cumin, garlic, lime juice and a pinch of sea salt. Mix well then put to one side.

Heat the ghee or butter in a large frying pan over a high heat. Add the chicken and stir-fry for 2 minutes. Then add the green beans, baby sweetcorn and sugar snap peas and stir-fry for a further 2 minutes.

Add the curry paste and cook for another minute. Add the broth and lime leaves and bring to the boil. Reduce the heat and add the arrowroot paste, stirring well. Simmer for 7 minutes.

Add the spinach and cook for 1 minute. Remove from the heat and add the basil leaves just before serving. Serve with basmati or other rice.

duck breast, orange blossom celeriac and shiitake

A truly delectable dish that uses orange blossom to give the signature fruity flavour synonymous with duck. The celeriac provides useful fibre for the microbiome. Shiitake, like other mushrooms, are an excellent prebiotic that helps to satiate our gut microbes, and their earthy flavour works beautifully alongside the richness of the duck.

serves 2

1 medium–large celeriac (approx. 750g), peeled and cut into 1cm chunks

2 free range duck breasts

3 tablespoons organic butter

½ teaspoon orange blossom water

80g shiitake mushrooms, sliced

1 tablespoon tamari

Sea salt and black pepper

Couple sprigs of marjoram or oregano, leaves picked

Extra virgin olive oil to serve

Preheat the oven to 200°C/Gas 6. Steam or boil the celeriac until tender.

Meanwhile, score the skin of the duck breasts in diagonal lines. Season with salt and pepper. Place the duck breasts skin side down in a cold non-stick frying pan. Place the pan over a medium heat and cook for 5–7 minutes until the skin is golden brown. Using tongs, turn the breasts over and seal on the other side for about a minute. Transfer the breasts, skin side up, to a rack in a roasting pan and roast for 15 minutes.

When the celeriac is cooked, drain and tip into a blender. Add 2 tablespoons of the butter, the orange blossom water, a pinch of salt and pepper and blend until smooth. You may need to stop and scrape or use your tamper to push the celeriac down. Leave in the blender so that it keeps its heat. By this point your duck should be ready, so remove from the oven and leave to rest for 10 minutes.

Heat the remaining tablespoon of butter in a frying pan over a medium heat. Add the sliced shiitake and fry for 5–6 minutes until golden. For the last 30 seconds, add the tamari.

Divide the celeriac purée between two plates and serve the mushrooms alongside. Slice the duck breasts horizontally into thin slices and lay on top of the celeriac. Sprinkle with fresh marjoram or oregano leaves and finish with a drizzle of olive oil.

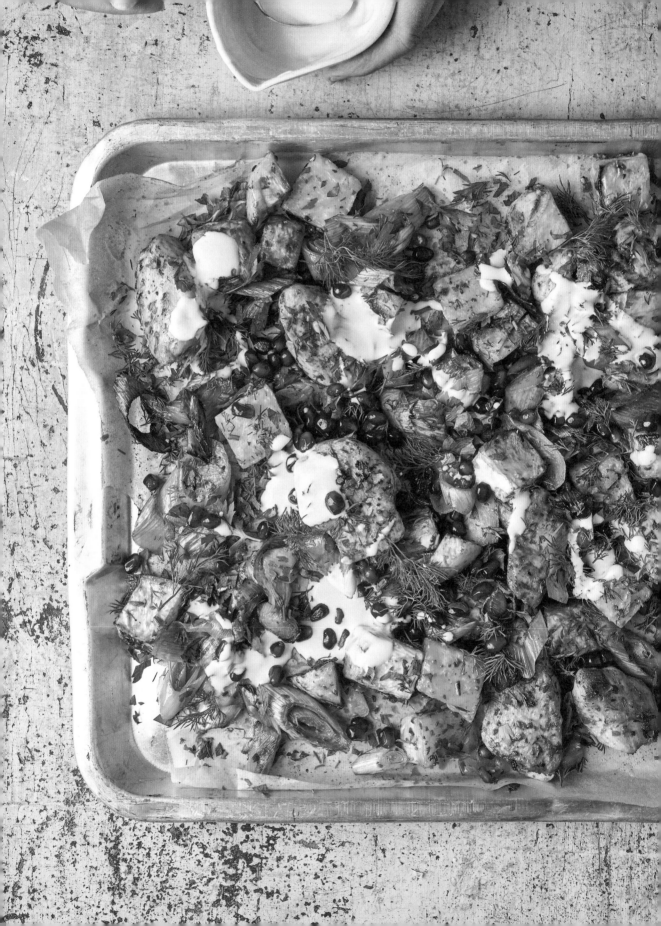

harissa chicken with lemon and pomegranate dressing

Dishes don't come much more restorative and nourishing than this. The flavours are amazing and it's so easy to make; you can sit back and relax while it cooks. Chicken is a good source of tryptophan, which is the precursor to 'happy' serotonin, while the celeriac and leeks offer abundant fibre – fuel for our microbes. With the bold flavours of harissa, jewel-like pomegranate seeds and vibrant herbs it's a delight for the senses, the mind and the microbiome.

serves 2

2 teaspoons harissa paste

2 tablespoons organic butter, melted

2 teaspoons ground cumin

1 teaspoon ground coriander

Juice of ½ lemon

½ teaspoon sea salt

2 organic free range chicken breasts, each sliced into 6 pieces

1 small–medium celeriac (about 450g), peeled and cut into 3.5cm cubes

2 leeks, sliced on the diagonal, around 1 cm thick

1 small bunch fresh flat-leaf parsley, roughly chopped

1 small bunch dill, roughly chopped

lemon and pomegranate dressing

2 tablespoons goats' or sheep's milk yogurt

Juice of ½ lemon

¼ teaspoon garlic-infused olive oil (or ½ crushed garlic clove and ¼ teaspoon extra virgin olive oil)

½ tablespoon filtered water

1 tablespoon pomegranate seeds

Mix together the harissa, butter, cumin, coriander, lemon juice and salt to create the marinade. Put the chicken in a large bowl, add the celeriac and leeks and pour over the marinade. Massage well and leave for at least 20 minutes to an hour.

Preheat the oven to 200°C/Gas 6. Line a large baking tray with baking parchment. Place the chicken, celeriac and leeks on the baking tray and bake for 40 minutes, tossing halfway through cooking time so that everything bakes evenly.

To make the dressing, combine the yogurt, lemon juice, garlic oil and water in a small bowl with a pinch of sea salt.

Remove the baking tray from the oven and sprinkle over the chopped herbs, haphazardly dollop over the dressing and top with the pomegranate seeds. You can serve at the table in the pan or divide between two plates.

wine pairing

Enjoy this dish with a white Assyrtiko or a Languedoc red such as Corbières, Minervois or St-Chinian.

rosemary beef stew and cauliflower champ

This glorious stew celebrates slow cooking and the anticipation of eating. Because this is slow cooked you can use less expensive, and potentially lesser used, cuts such as shin or blade that help us to be more mindful of the food we are buying. Organic meat provides essential omega 3 fatty acids that are important for the health of our gut and brain, and the cauliflower champ gives a nice boost of fibre for our microbes.

serves 4

450g organic grass-fed beef cuts – I like to use shin but you can use any stewing cut

1 tablespoon organic butter

3 leeks, sliced on the diagonal, around 1 cm thick

1 garlic clove, crushed or finely sliced

300ml organic beef bone broth

150ml red wine

1 tablespoon finely chopped fresh rosemary

3–4 tablespoons Parmesan, grated

Sea salt and black pepper

cauliflower champ

1 small cauliflower, cut into florets

½ tablespoon organic butter

¼ teaspoon mustard powder

1 teaspoon apple cider vinegar

Preheat the oven to 170°C/Gas 3. Cut the beef into chunks, about 5cm square. Season with a generous couple of pinches of sea salt and pepper. Heat the butter in a large flameproof casserole (with a lid) over a medium heat and add the beef. Cook for a couple of minutes, turning occasionally until nicely browned all over. Transfer to a large bowl.

Add the leeks to the casserole and cook for 5 minutes. Add the garlic and cook for a further minute. Return the meat to the pan along with the broth, wine and rosemary. Bring to the boil and then cover the pan with the lid and put into the oven for 1½ hours.

While the beef is cooking, prepare the champ. Boil or steam the cauliflower for 10 minutes. Place in a blender with the butter, mustard and vinegar and blend to a purée.

Sprinkle the grated Parmesan over the stew and serve with the cauliflower champ on the side. You can also serve with a green vegetable such as broccoli or green beans.

miso and honey-glazed chicken with coriander and sesame carrots

Miso, honey and ginger provide a rich glaze for the chicken thighs and create a gold medal-winning flavour sensation. I use thighs with the skin on as they are packed full of healthy fats to help support the brain and gut.

serves 2

120g unpasteurised sweet white miso paste

15g organic butter, softened

½ teaspoon ground ginger

1 teaspoon raw honey

2 tablespoons coconut aminos (or 1 tablespoon tamari and 1 tablespoon mirin)

Black pepper

4 organic free range chicken thighs (about 500g)

1 tablespoon sesame seeds

coriander and sesame carrots

175g baby carrots, washed or scrubbed, but not peeled

2 tablespoons roughly chopped fresh coriander

2 teaspoons sesame oil

Sea salt

Line a baking tray with baking parchment. Mix the miso, butter, ginger, honey, coconut aminos and a generous pinch of black pepper to form a paste. Massage into the chicken thighs, place on the baking tray and set aside for 30 minutes.

Preheat the oven to 180°C/Gas 4.

Place the chicken in the oven and roast for 35 minutes. Leave to rest for 5 minutes.

Towards the end of the chicken cooking time, lightly boil or steam the carrots for 5–10 minutes until just tender. Drain and place in a bowl then mix through the coriander, sesame oil and a pinch of sea salt.

Divide the carrots between two plates, add the chicken and sprinkle with sesame seeds.

spicy marinated chicken with garlic greens and ginger satay

Inspired by my neighbourhood and the Notting Hill carnival I decided to create this dish with Caribbean style flavours. After the celebrations are over, sitting down to savour this can restore some peace and tranquillity to the body and mind. Chicken is one of the highest sources of tryptophan, which helps support mood and the sleep–wake cycle, while the greens provide vitamin B6 and magnesium – also important for sleep. Perfect after-party food.

serves 2

spicy chicken

1½ teaspoons ground allspice

1 teaspoon onion powder

½ teaspoon ground cinnamon

Pinch grated nutmeg

Pinch black pepper

Pinch cayenne

2 organic free range chicken breasts

1 tablespoon organic butter

Sea salt

thyme carrots

150g small carrots

1 tablespoon organic butter, melted

3–4 sprigs fresh thyme

ginger satay

2½ tablespoons unsweetened smooth peanut butter

1 tablespoon tomato paste

1 tablespoon coconut aminos

¼ teaspoon garlic powder

¼ teaspoon ground ginger

Pinch black pepper

Squeeze lime juice

50ml filtered water

For the spicy chicken, mix all the spices, rub over the chicken and set aside for 30 minutes

Preheat the oven to 200°C/Gas 6. Line a baking tray with baking parchment.

For the thyme carrots, wash the carrots, brush and trim if you need but keep the skin on. Place on the baking tray and drizzle over the butter. Remove some of the thyme leaves and scatter over the carrots then add the whole sprigs. Roast for 40 minutes.

In a large saucepan with a lid, melt 1 tablespoon of butter over a medium–high heat and sear the chicken for 1 minute. Turn the chicken over and turn the heat down to low. Cover with the lid and cook for 10 minutes. Remove from the heat but keep the lid on and leave the chicken to sit for a further 10 minutes.

To make the satay, mix all of the ingredients together in a small bowl.

When the chicken is cooked, remove from the pan and leave to rest for 5 minutes.

garlic greens
1 tablespoon organic butter
1 small red onion, finely sliced
1 garlic clove
100g collard greens, chard or spinach
½ teaspoon chilli flakes

Cook the greens in the same pan in which you cooked the chicken, so that you get all of the lovely juices. Melt the butter, add the onion and garlic and stir-fry for 2 minutes. Then add the greens and chilli flakes and fry for another minute.

Serve the greens with the carrots alongside. Slice the chicken on the diagonal and place on the greens. Spoon over the satay sauce and finish with a pinch of sea salt.

beef tagliata, Parmesan and rocket

Simple, yet incredibly delicious. This is all about the quality of the ingredients. Retired dairy beef is exactly what it implies: it is from cows formerly used for milk production, making it a more sustainable choice. It also has a lot of marbling that enhances the flavour. If you're looking for a stress-free supper, this dish is all about fuss-free enjoyment.

serves 2

2 organic dairy beef sirloin steaks (see shopping guide) or organic grass-fed steaks
1 tablespoon extra virgin olive oil, plus extra for brushing
2 generous handfuls rocket
1 tablespoon aged balsamic vinegar
30g Parmesan, shaved
Sea salt and black pepper

Remove the steaks from the fridge and allow to come to room temperature. Season and brush with a little olive oil.

Heat a griddle pan (or a frying pan if you don't have a griddle) over a very high heat. Sear the steaks on each side for 2 minutes (if you like them rare) or 3 minutes or longer if you prefer well done. Remove from the pan and leave to rest for at least 5 minutes. Then slice into strips about 1cm thick.

Arrange the rocket on two plates, lay the steak across the leaves, drizzle with the balsamic and olive oil and finish with Parmesan shavings.

pistachio-crusted lamb cutlets, artichokes and mint

Combining ingredients and flavours to lip-smacking effect, this delicious dish will satisfy your microbiome and mind as well as your taste buds. Organic lamb is a good source of omega 3 essential fatty acids, important for the health of the brain and gut. Artichokes provide prebiotic fibre to 'feed' your microbes and they perfectly complement the pistachio and lamb in this dish. Serve this with buttery new potatoes or wild rice.

serves 2

30g shelled pistachios, ground (I use a coffee/spice grinder for this but you can very finely chop instead)

½ teaspoon mustard powder

1 tablespoon fresh lemon juice

1 teaspoon extra virgin olive oil, plus approx. 2 teaspoons to sauté the artichokes

6 organic grass-fed lamb cutlets

200g cooked artichokes (ideally source those in glass jars)

Small handful fresh mint leaves, roughly torn

Sea salt and black pepper

In a small bowl, mix together the ground pistachios and mustard powder and season with sea salt and black pepper. Add the lemon juice and olive oil and stir to form a paste. Press the paste evenly over one side of the lamb cutlets and set aside for 20–30 minutes.

Preheat the oven to 200°C/Gas 6. Line a baking tray with foil.

Heat a large frying pan over a medium heat and brown the underside of the lamb cutlets (the side without the pistachio crust). Then place on the baking tray, crust side up, and roast for 10 minutes. Remove from the oven and leave to rest for 5 minutes.

Meanwhile, drain the artichokes, pat dry on kitchen paper and cut into thin slices. Heat a little olive oil in a pan and lightly sauté the artichokes to warm through and give them a bit of colour. Remove from the heat and toss with the mint leaves.

Divide the artichokes between two plates and lay the lamb cutlets alongside.

wine pairing

Try a flavoursome red such as Rioja Reserva or a wine from Cabernet Franc grapes, such as Chinon, Bourgueil or Saumur–Champigny.

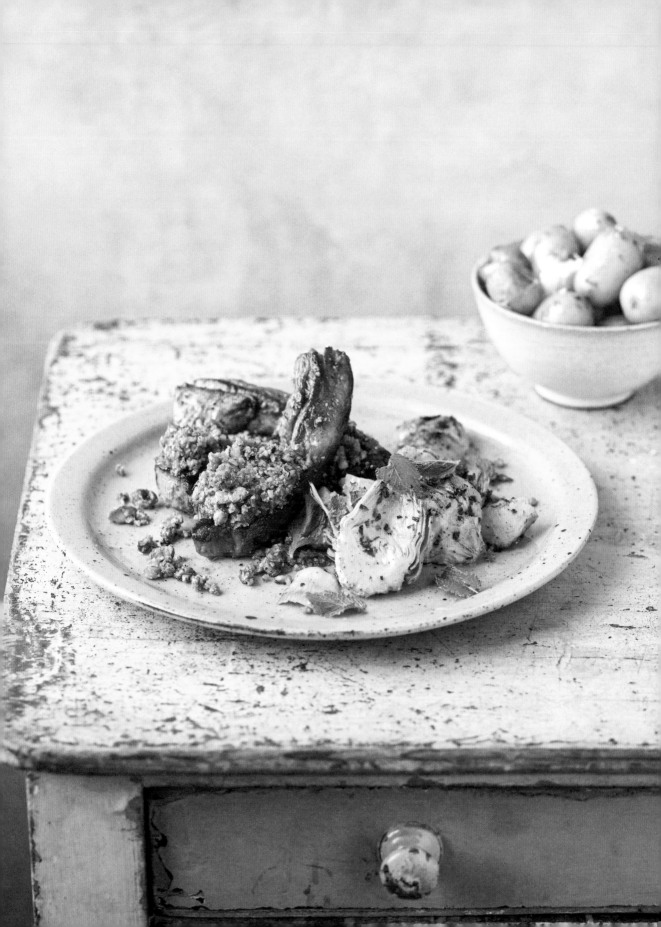

za'atar spiced lamb burger with broccoli and romesco sauce

Za'atar is a fragrant mix of herbs and toasted sesame seeds that goes wonderfully with lamb. Organic grass-fed meat is a good source of the omega 3 essential fatty acids that are so important for many reasons, including the health of our gut and brain. The spicy broccoli and red pepper sauce are colourful accompaniments that provide plenty of polyphenols to satisfy your microbiome.

serves 2

250g organic grass-fed lamb mince

4 teaspoons za'atar

romesco sauce

2 red peppers, about 180g

25g flaked almonds, toasted

2 tablespoons tomato paste

¼ teaspoon garlic powder (or ½ fresh garlic clove)

2 teaspoons smoked paprika

1 tablespoon extra virgin olive oil

1 tablespoon fresh lemon juice

Pinch sea salt

broccoli

250g tenderstem broccoli

¼ teaspoon chilli flakes

1 teaspoon olive oil

Preheat the oven to 200°C/Gas 6. Line a baking tray with baking parchment. Cut the peppers in half lengthways, remove the seeds and stalks and then slice into strips. Place on the baking tray and roast for 25 minutes.

In a large bowl, mix the lamb and the za'atar, using your hands. Divide into four burgers and leave to rest.

Once the peppers are soft, remove them from the oven and set aside. Turn the oven down to 190°C/Gas 5. Line a baking tray with foil, lay the burgers on the foil and cook for 25 minutes.

Meanwhile, make the romesco sauce. Place the cooked peppers with all of the other sauce ingredients in a food processor and blitz until you get a thick sauce.

Once the burgers are cooked, remove from the oven and leave to rest. To cook the broccoli, bring a pan of water to the boil, add the broccoli and boil for 2 minutes. Take the pan off the heat, drain the broccoli and put it back in the pan with the chilli flakes and olive oil. Stir to mix evenly.

Serve two lamb burgers per person, with the broccoli alongside and 2–3 tablespoons (or more if you like) of the romesco sauce.

tip

If you have any sauce left over, store it in a small container in the fridge. It is delicious with eggs and sourdough for brunch the next day.

lamb neck fillet, courgettes and salsa verde

Lamb neck is one of the more unusual cuts: in this recipe you can replace it with cutlets or leg steaks but using alternative cuts such as neck can help us to consume our meat more sustainably and mindfully. Organic lamb is a great source of anti-inflammatory omega-3s and other fats that can help to support the brain as well as the gut. The anchovies in the salsa verde also provide an extra boost of omega-3s.

serves 2

250g organic grass-fed lamb neck, cut into 5cm chunks

1 teaspoon dried oregano

Extra virgin olive oil

2 courgettes (ideally one green and one yellow)

Generous handful spinach leaves

1 tablespoon balsamic vinegar

Sea salt and black pepper

Seasonal edible flowers to garnish (optional)

salsa verde

3 anchovy fillets, drained

1 tablespoon capers, rinsed and drained

¼ teaspoon mustard powder

1 garlic clove, crushed

1 tablespoon fresh lemon juice

4 tablespoons extra virgin olive oil

Small handful fresh parsley

Small handful fresh basil

Remove the lamb from the fridge and allow to come to room temperature. Season with the oregano and a couple of pinches of sea salt and pepper and rub with a little olive oil.

To make the salsa verde, pat dry the anchovy fillets and capers with kitchen paper. Place all the salsa verde ingredients in a food processor, add a good pinch of salt and pepper and process to make a thick sauce. Transfer to a small bowl and place in the fridge.

Cut the courgettes lengthways into quarters and then into 2–3cm chunks. Put to one side while you cook the lamb.

Heat a large frying pan over a high heat. Add the lamb chunks and cook for 3–5 minutes, turning so that they cook evenly. Transfer to a plate to rest.

While the lamb is resting drizzle a little olive oil into the pan and add the courgettes. Stir-fry for around 3 minutes. Add the spinach and balsamic and fry for a further 1 minute.

Serve the courgettes and spinach with the lamb on top and drizzle over the salsa verde. Garnish with the flowers if using.

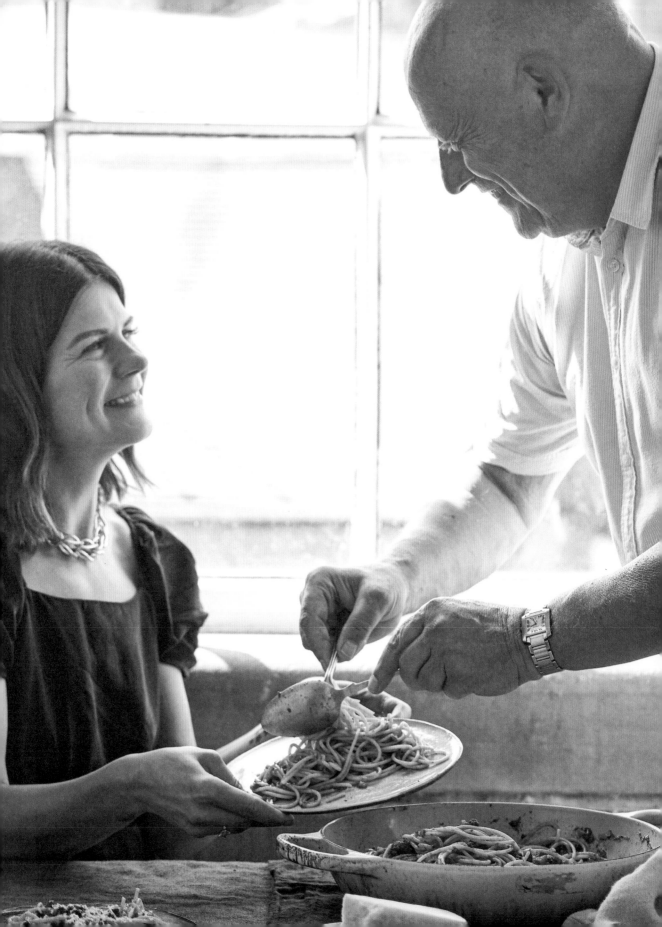

dad's spag bol

A riff on an age-old family fave. As kids we used to be transfixed watching my dad meticulously chopping the carrots, tomatoes and celery in his signature perfectionist style. I have to admit my version is nowhere near as neat. However, the result is nothing short of magical. The veggies provide fibre and the organic meat and chicken livers boast many nutritional benefits, including omega 3 fatty acids, vitamin A and plentiful amounts of B vitamins, which are important for the gut and the brain. This dish is altogether nourishing and perfect for family togetherness time.

serves 4

2 tablespoons organic butter

1 onion, finely chopped

1 carrot, finely diced

1 celery stalk, finely chopped

225g organic grass-fed beef mince

100g organic chicken livers, finely chopped

350g tomatoes, finely chopped

2 tablespoons tomato paste

150ml red wine

300ml organic beef bone broth

1 bay leaf

1 teaspoon dried oregano

1 teaspoon dried basil

½ teaspoon sea salt

300g spaghetti

Finely grated Parmesan to serve

Heat the butter in a saucepan over a medium heat. Add the onion, carrot and celery and cook for 8–10 minutes, stirring occasionally. Add the minced beef and cook, stirring, for about 10 minutes or until the meat is well browned.

Add the chicken livers, tomatoes, tomato paste, wine, broth, bay leaf, oregano, basil and salt. Reduce the heat to low, cover the pan and simmer for 1 hour.

Cook the spaghetti until al dente. Drain and divide between four bowls. Then divide the sauce between the bowls, removing the bay leaf when you come across it. Finish with a generous handful of Parmesan in each bowl.

tip

If anyone in your family is sensitive to gluten, look for gluten-free alternatives to spaghetti, made from buckwheat or rice flour.

wine pairing

This calls for a rich and juicy Italian red such as Sangiovese, Rosso di Montalcino or Barbera.

five-spice pork burgers on chilli and garlic greens with coconut onion rings

These vibrantly flavoured burgers taste amazing and are visually enticing too. What's more, the sweet and crunchy onion rings provide a feast for the microbiome, since onion is a prebiotic food and coconut flour a good source of fibre. The greens provide additional antioxidants and fibre for both brain and gut. If you like, serve with Miso Slaw (page 119).

serves 4

400g organic outdoor-reared pork mince

1 garlic clove, crushed

¼ teaspoon ground ginger

1 teaspoon Chinese five spice powder

1 tablespoon coconut aminos (or 1 teaspoon tamari and 1 teaspoon mirin or rice wine vinegar)

Sea salt and black pepper

onion rings

1 red onion, peeled

2 tablespoons coconut flour

1 organic egg

1 teaspoon arrowroot

1 tablespoon desiccated coconut

chilli greens

1 tablespoon coconut oil

200g tenderstem broccoli, trimmed

1 red chilli, deseeded and finely sliced

2 garlic cloves, finely sliced

200g pak choi, trimmed

1 tablespoon coconut aminos (or 1 teaspoon tamari and 1 teaspoon mirin or rice wine vinegar)

Preheat the oven to 200°C/Gas 6. Line a baking tray with foil.

In a large bowl, mix the pork with the garlic, spices, coconut aminos and a pinch of salt and pepper. Shape into four patties, about 1cm thick. Leave to rest while you prepare the onion rings.

Cut the onion into 3mm thick slices then separate each layer of the onion into rings. Set up three stations for coating the onion rings. Put 1 tablespoon of the coconut flour on a sheet of baking paper or a tray. Whisk the egg in a bowl. In another bowl combine the arrowroot, desiccated coconut, 1 tablespoon of coconut flour and a pinch of sea salt and mix well. Line a baking tray with baking parchment. Dust the onion rings in the coconut flour, dip briefly in the egg and then lightly coat in the coconut and arrowroot batter. Place on the baking tray and put to one side.

Place the burgers on the foil-lined baking tray and bake for 15 minutes. Turn the burgers over and return to the oven. Put the onion rings on a higher shelf in the oven and bake for 20 minutes.

About 5 minutes before the burgers and onion rings are ready, start to cook the chilli greens. In a large frying pan, heat the coconut oil then add the broccoli and a splash of water and stir-fry over a high heat for 2–3 minutes. Add the chilli and garlic and stir-fry for 1 minute. Then add the pak choi and coconut aminos and stir-fry for a further minute.

Divide the greens between four plates. Place the burgers on top and serve with the onion rings.

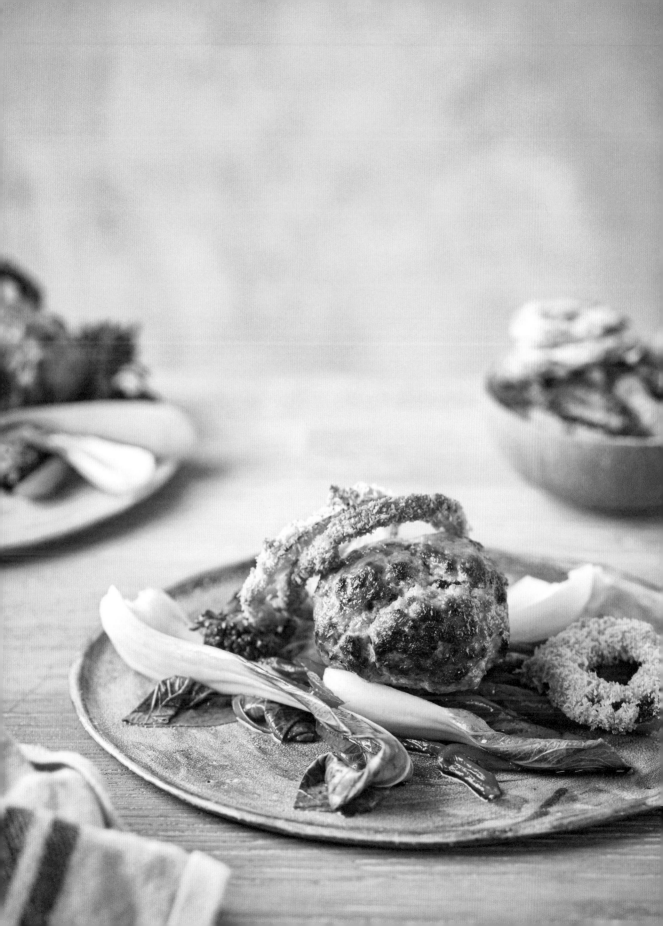

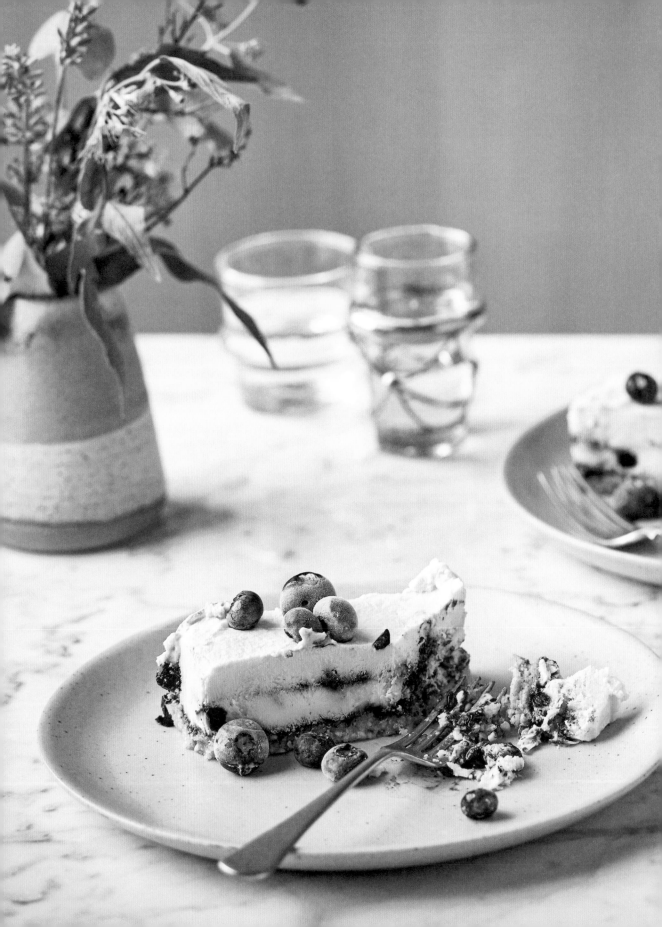

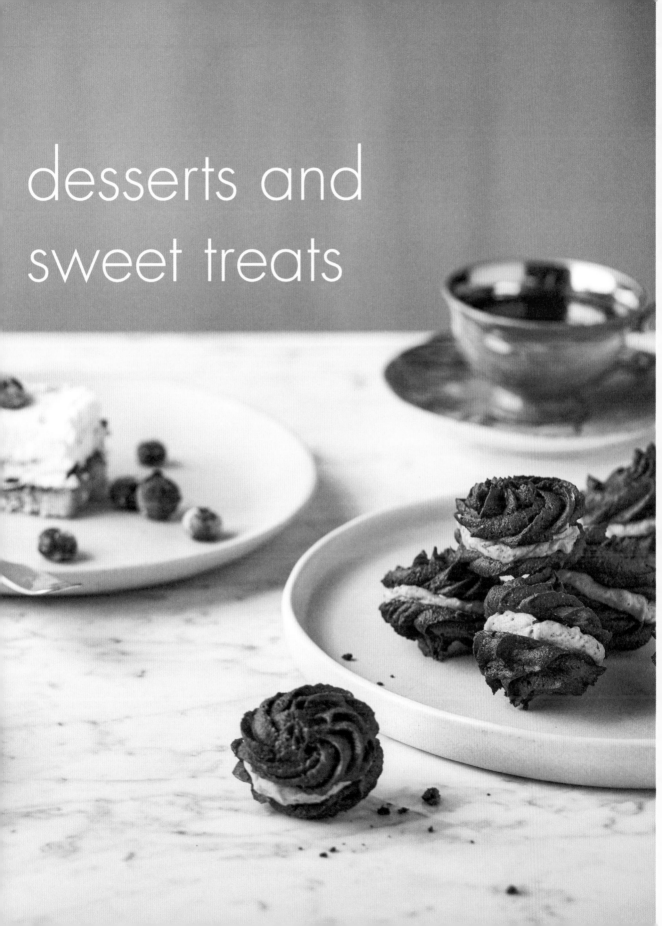

desserts and
sweet treats

seasonal fruit fools

These versatile fruit fools can be varied according to the fruits that are ripe and ready. If you use apples, stewing them releases more of the pectin, a type of fibre that feeds the beneficial microbes in our gut. On the other hand, using fresh uncooked fruit retains more of the vitamin C and includes other types of fibre, to provide diversity for our microbiome. Ricotta is made from the whey left over after making cheese; like other cheeses it contains bacteria that are believed to be beneficial for our gut. A simple yet sumptuous dessert that can be served as a breakfast too.

serves 2

150g ricotta, drained

1 teaspoon honey

½ teaspoon vanilla extract

150g seasonal fruit

2 tablespoons filtered water (optional)

1 tablespoon chopped nuts (see tip)

Put the ricotta, honey and vanilla in a bowl and vigorously whisk together. Place in the fridge.

If you are using firm fruit such as apples or pears, core and cut them into roughly 4cm chunks and place in a large saucepan. Add the water and place over a low heat. Simmer for about 10 minutes or until the fruit is soft. Leave to cool.

If you are using soft fruit such as peaches, nectarines or strawberries, simply stone as necessary and slice the fruit.

In two small jars or tumblers, start with a layer of half the fruit, then add a layer of the whipped ricotta, add the remaining fruit and finish with the remaining ricotta. Sprinkle the chopped nuts on top.

tip

I recommend almonds with apples, hazelnuts with pears, pistachios with apricots, peaches or nectarines, and pecans with strawberries, but play around and have fun with flavour combos.

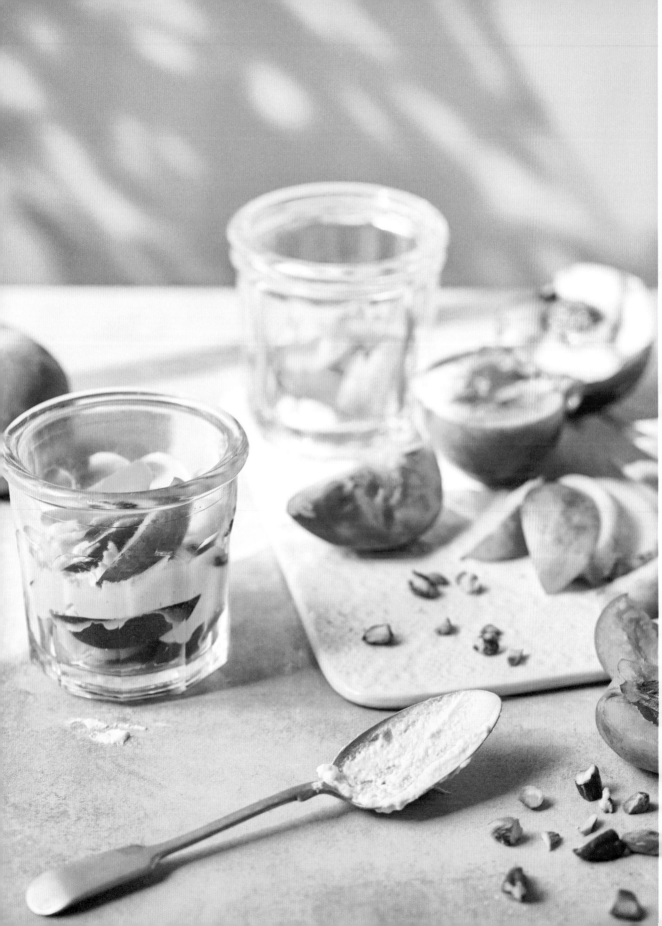

positive chocolate pot de crème

Just looking at one of these little chocolate pots sparks joy. And once you gleefully tuck in, your taste buds will be rewarded. Chocolate has myriad positive things going for it in terms of antioxidants and polyphenols that help to support both gut and brain health, so let's leave it at that and just enjoy.

serves 1

100g ricotta
25g unsweetened cocoa powder
1½ teaspoons honey
½ teaspoon vanilla extract

Place all the ingredients in a bowl and whisk until thick and smooth. Transfer to a small glass or espresso cup and store in the fridge until ready to serve.

tip

To make a vegan version, replace the ricotta with silken tofu and the honey with maple syrup.

---

baobab-ana n-ice cream

Baobab has a delicious citrusy flavour, is a good source of antioxidants and, combined with bananas, provides a double helping of fibre for your microbiome. Blending frozen bananas is a simple way to make ice cream – or serve this unfrozen as a creamy topping for porridge or yogurt.

makes 3–4 servings

5 small or 4 medium ripe bananas
200ml (1 small tin) full fat coconut milk
50g baobab powder, plus extra for dusting (optional)
2 tablespoons raw honey

Thinly slice the bananas and freeze for at least 2 hours.

Put all the ingredients into a powerful blender and pulse on high until smooth and very thick. You can eat it straight away if you prefer a soft consistency, or make it firmer by transferring to a container and freezing for an hour. Dust with extra baobab powder before serving. Store in the freezer or the fridge for up to 2 days.

Midas ice cream

This ice cream really does have the Midas touch, with its rich golden colour and mix of heady spices. Saffron is associated with neuroprotective benefits, possibly linked to its high antioxidant content. This recipe uses arrowroot rather than the traditional eggs to bind, as I find it's easier to get an even consistency. Arrowroot is also a source of resistant starch, which your microbes will appreciate, and using this instead of eggs means that the recipe is suitable for those following an exclusively plant-based diet.

makes approx. 600g

125g almond butter
300ml filtered water
60g coconut butter
75g coconut sugar
50g honey
2 teaspoons ground turmeric
½ teaspoon ground cardamom
Seeds from 1 vanilla pod or ½ teaspoon vanilla extract
Generous pinch saffron strands
Pinch black pepper
1½ teaspoons arrowroot
3–4 ice cubes

Place all the ingredients in a blender and blend until smooth. Transfer to a large bowl and freeze.

After 45 minutes, remove from the freezer and whisk. Return to the freezer. Repeat this every 30 minutes until you have whisked the part-frozen mixture four times. Your ice cream is done! Store in a freezerproof container until ready to serve.

note

If you are lucky enough to own an ice-cream maker then after blending you can transfer the liquid to your machine and leave it to do its thing!

salted liquorice ice cream

Food can evoke many memories and help us to express our appreciation of our shared experiences with other people. For me, this recipe sings for my brother because he absolutely loved liquorice. I decided to create both dairy and non-dairy versions so that everyone can enjoy this sumptuous and memorable dessert.

makes approx. 600g

300ml Jersey or Guernsey double cream

250ml Jersey or Guernsey full fat milk

100g coconut sugar

2 tablespoons liquorice powder

3 tablespoons maple syrup

1 teaspoon vanilla extract

2 teaspoons arrowroot powder

2 generous pinches sea salt

non-dairy option

300ml unsweetened almond milk

60g coconut butter

100g coconut sugar

2 tablespoons liquorice powder

3 tablespoons maple syrup

1 teaspoon vanilla extract

2 teaspoons arrowroot powder

2 generous pinches sea salt

Use either the first list of ingredients or the non-dairy option. Place all the ingredients in a blender and blend until smooth. Transfer to a large bowl and freeze.

After 45 minutes, remove from the freezer and whisk. Return to the freezer. Repeat this every 30 minutes until you have whisked the part-frozen mixture four times. Leave in the freezer to set for a further 2 hours.

note

If you are lucky enough to own an ice-cream maker then after blending you can transfer the liquid to your machine and leave it to do its thing!

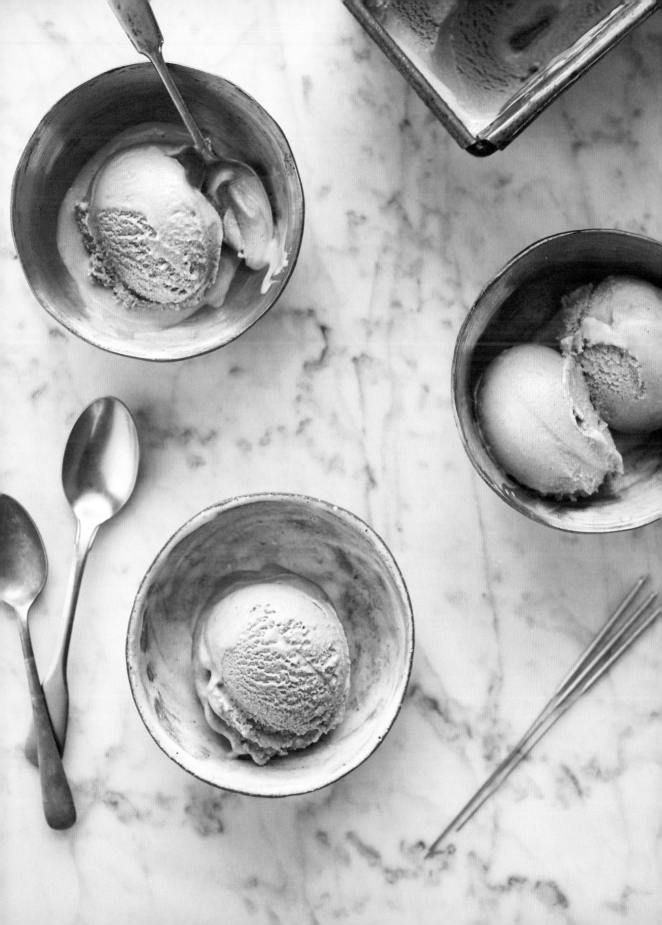

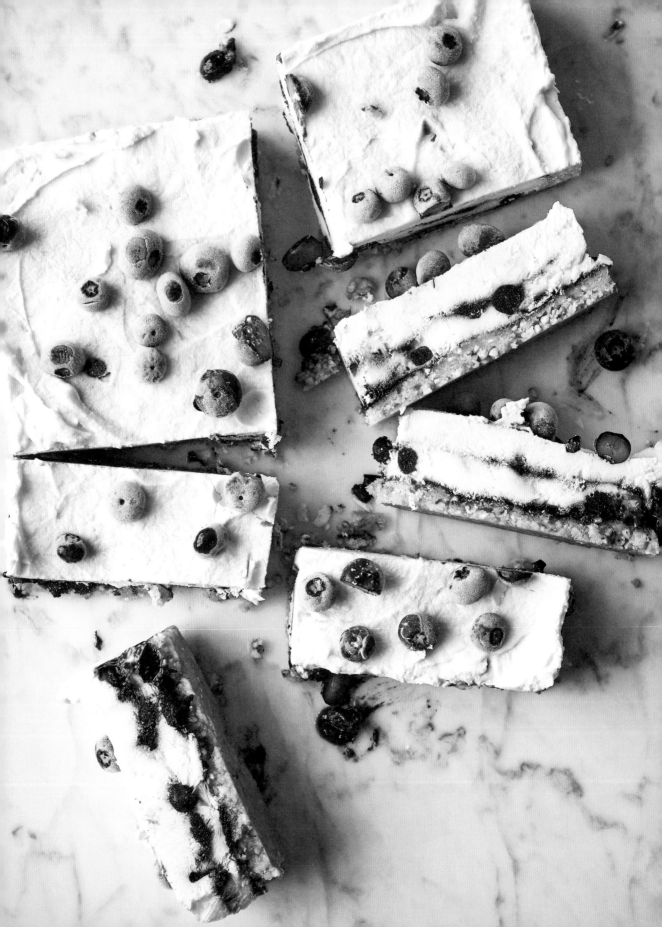

blueberry swirl cheesecake

This cheesecake features both ricotta and mascarpone cheese to provide a good source of beneficial bacteria to support overall gut health. The base is made from fibre-rich buckwheat and creamy macadamia nuts that together can have a prebiotic 'feeding' effect on the microbiome.

serves 8

300g blueberries

3½ tablespoons honey

50g buckwheat groats (ideally sprouted)

100g macadamia nuts

Sea salt

250g mascarpone

250g ricotta

Set aside 100g of the blueberries for the topping. Put the remaining blueberries in a saucepan with ½ tablespoon of the honey over a low–medium heat for 6–8 minutes until the blueberries begin to break down, leaving some of the blueberries intact. Transfer to a small bowl, place to one side.

Put the buckwheat, macadamia nuts and a pinch of sea salt in a food processor and pulse to a fine crumb texture. Add 2 tablespoons of the honey and pulse again to combine. Use a 15cm square baking tin, ideally with a removable base, or line a 15cm square tin with baking paper so that you can easily lift out the cheesecake. Press the buckwheat mixture evenly into the tin. Put in the fridge for about 1 hour to firm up.

Put the mascarpone, ricotta and 1 tablespoon of honey into a large bowl and beat until thick and evenly combined.

Remove the base from the fridge. Spread half the blueberry mixture evenly over the buckwheat base. Then add half of the mascarpone mixture and spread evenly. Add the remaining blueberry mixture and then finally the remaining mascarpone mixture. Using a skewer, swirl into the cream to create a ripple effect. Smooth the top and sprinkle over the reserved blueberries. Put into the freezer for 3 hours. (You can leave it for longer but you will need to allow 1 hour for the cheesecake to defrost.) To serve, cut into eight slices.

salted caramel apples

This glorious combination is really easy to make. Stewing the apples releases more of their pectin, a unique type of fibre that helps to 'feed' our microbes so that they can produce anti-inflammatory substances that help to maintain a healthy gut and brain. These apples are great as a dessert with yogurt or whipped ricotta and a little honey, or on porridge or overnight oats.

serves 2

200g apples
2–4 tablespoons filtered water

caramel sauce
2 tablespoons almond butter
2 tablespoons coconut sugar
Squeeze lemon juice
3–4 tablespoons filtered water
Sea salt

Do not peel the apples, just chop them into 5cm cubes, discarding the cores. Place in a large saucepan, add a small amount of filtered water (about 2 tablespoons) to cover the base of the pan and bring to the boil over a medium heat. Reduce the heat and simmer for 10 minutes until soft. You may need to add a little more water if the pan becomes dry, but add it little by little if needed.

Meanwhile, to make the caramel sauce, combine in a small bowl the almond butter, coconut sugar, lemon juice, 3–4 tablespoons filtered water, as needed to make a smooth sauce, and a couple of generous pinches of sea salt. Drizzle the sauce over the apples or serve on the side.

almond and anise gooey cookies

Once you have made these cookies you will come back to them time and time again. Brimming with the flavour of aniseed and ingredients that are bursting with fibre they're a treat for your taste buds and microbes. So take a precious moment in your day to sit and be present, enjoying your gooey cookie with Sweet Dreams Milk or a Maca Mocha (see page 193).

makes 18 cookies

180g chestnut flour
125g ground almonds
45g coconut sugar
1 teaspoon vanilla extract
1 teaspoon ground star anise
1 teaspoon fennel seeds
Sea salt
3 tablespoons almond butter
200ml (1 small tin) full fat coconut milk
100ml filtered water
100g flaked almonds

Preheat the oven to 180°C/Gas 4. Line two baking trays with baking parchment.

Place the chestnut flour, ground almonds, coconut sugar, vanilla, star anise, fennel seeds and a pinch of sea salt into a food processor. Pulse until combined. Add the almond butter and gradually add the coconut milk and water, pulsing to create a dough. Add the flaked almonds and pulse briefly but keep some texture.

Using an ice-cream scoop, scoop the mixture onto the lined baking trays and bake for 25 minutes. Transfer to a wire rack to cool completely.

chocolate and hazelnut Viennese whirls

These whirls taste amazing and are a treat for the microbiome. Chestnut flour and hazelnut butter are rich in fibre, and cocoa powder is very high in antioxidants: together, these foods help to support and feed the microbes in your gut. This in turn can help to support mood, so grab the opportunity for an uplifting moment in your day with these joyful little treats. What's more they are gluten-free and plant-based.

makes approx. 12 whirls

160g chestnut flour
25g unsweetened cocoa powder
100g coconut sugar
120g smooth hazelnut butter
200ml filtered water

filling

50g coconut butter (or creamed coconut)
½ teaspoon vanilla extract
50ml filtered water
20g smooth hazelnut butter
10g coconut sugar

First make the filling: put the coconut butter, vanilla and water in a small saucepan over a very low heat and stir gently until creamy. Transfer to a mixing bowl, add the hazelnut butter and coconut sugar and stir to combine, then whisk until thick. Place in the freezer for 10 minutes.

Preheat the oven to 180°C/Gas 4. Line two large baking trays with baking parchment.

Sift the chestnut flour and cocoa powder into a large bowl. Add the coconut sugar, hazelnut butter and water and mix until thick and smooth. Transfer the mixture into a piping bag with a 1cm star piping tip. Pipe the mixture onto the baking trays to make 26 x 4.5cm circles. Bake for 20 minutes. Leave to cool.

Sandwich the biscuits with a generous teaspoon of the filling.

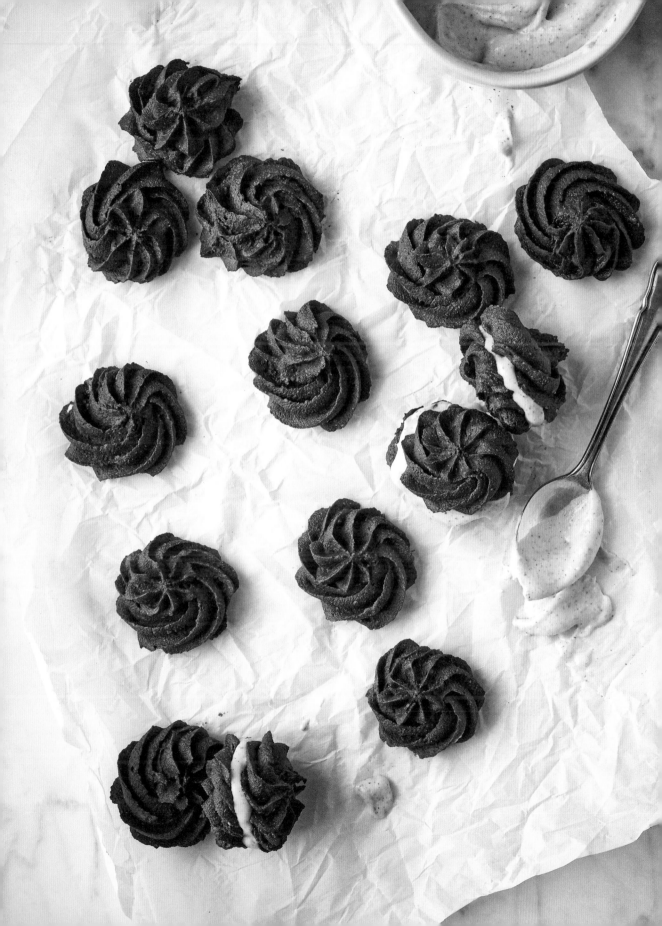

tiger nut truffles

Perfect for a little something after a meal, these simple truffles are a win–win for your microbiome and taste buds. Tiger nuts are actually mini tubers (not nuts) and are high in fibre and resistant starch, providing a veritable feast for your microbes. And because tiger nuts are naturally sweet, only a hint of honey is needed.

makes approx. 25 truffles

125g tiger nut flour or powder
40g unsweetened cocoa powder
20g ground almonds
3 tablespoons tahini
1 tablespoon sumac
30g coconut butter
2 teaspoons honey
100ml filtered water
3 tablespoons sesame seeds

Place the tiger nut flour or powder, cocoa powder, ground almonds, tahini, sumac, coconut butter and honey into a food processor. Pulse for a minute until fully combined. Slowly add the water to make a thick sticky mixture.

Place the sesame seeds in a small bowl. To make your truffles, take a generous pinch of the mixture and roll into a small ball, around 2–3cm diameter. Roll in the sesame seeds to coat evenly and put on a plate. Repeat until you have used all the mixture. Place the balls in the fridge and leave them to set for at least an hour. They will keep for 3–4 days.

matcha marzipan bars with coconut cream drizzle

These are perfect when you want to take a moment out of your day to enjoy a bit of peace and quiet. Matcha is high in antioxidants that can help to mitigate the effects of stress and provide support to both the gut and the brain. Because this recipe is based on almonds it also provides some fibre and is suitable for those who prefer to avoid wheat or gluten flours. Making these is a pleasure, as they require minimum equipment and effort with bountiful rewards.

makes 14 bars

100g ground almonds
50g coconut sugar
1 teaspoon matcha
½ teaspoon almond extract
1 tablespoon almond butter
2 tablespoons filtered water

coconut cream topping
30g coconut butter
½ teaspoon vanilla extract
2 tablespoons filtered water

Put the ground almonds, coconut sugar, matcha, almond extract, almond butter and water into a bowl and mix with a spoon to make a dough. Roll the dough into a log about 4cm thick and 19cm long. Put on a plate and into the freezer for an hour.

Cut the log into 1cm thick slices: you should be able to make around 14 slices. Turn onto their flat sides and arrange on the plate.

For the topping, melt the coconut butter, vanilla and water in a small saucepan over a low heat. Drizzle evenly over the slices and put them back in the freezer for 30 minutes until the coconut cream has set.

Transfer to the fridge until ready to eat. They will keep for up to 2–3 days.

pistachio, cardamom and fennel seed biscotti

It is part of British culture to believe that most situations can be resolved over a cuppa and a bickie, and I created these biscotti for the same reason. The combination of pistachios and almonds gives an Italian-inspired twist but also provides rich amounts of fibre for your microbiome. With the calmative properties of fennel seeds you'll find it very hard to feel stressed while enjoying one of these ... preferably with your favourite cuppa.

makes 20 biscotti

100g shelled pistachios

75g ground almonds

30g coconut flour, plus
1 tablespoon to flour the surface

2 teaspoons ground cardamom

2 teaspoons fennel seeds

1 teaspoon bicarbonate of soda

100g almond butter

3 tablespoons coconut butter

1 teaspoon vanilla extract

1 teaspoon almond extract

2 tablespoons apple cider vinegar

5 tablespoons maple syrup

100ml unsweetened almond milk

Preheat the oven to 170°C/Gas 3. Line a baking tray with baking parchment.

Place the pistachios in a food processor and pulse for around 30 seconds to break into smaller pieces: you want to keep some texture so avoid over-processing. Add the ground almonds, coconut flour, cardamom, fennel seeds and bicarbonate of soda. Pulse a few times to combine.

Add the almond butter, coconut butter, vanilla and almond extracts, apple cider vinegar and maple syrup. Pulse to combine. The mixture should start to stick at this point. Gradually add the milk to form a dough.

Sprinkle your work surface with coconut flour and tip the dough onto the surface. Divide it into two equal pieces and shape each half into a rectangle about 8cm wide by 2cm thick. Place on the lined baking tray and bake for 25 minutes.

Remove from the oven and leave to cool on the baking tray for 10 minutes. Turn the oven down to 150°C/Gas 2. After they have cooled for 10 minutes, cut the rectangles into 3cm thick slices using a serrated knife (approximately 10 slices per rectangle). Return to the oven and bake for 10 minutes, then turn and bake on the other side for a further 10 minutes.

Remove from the oven and leave to cool completely. Store in the fridge (gives extra crunch!) or in an airtight container for up to 5 days.

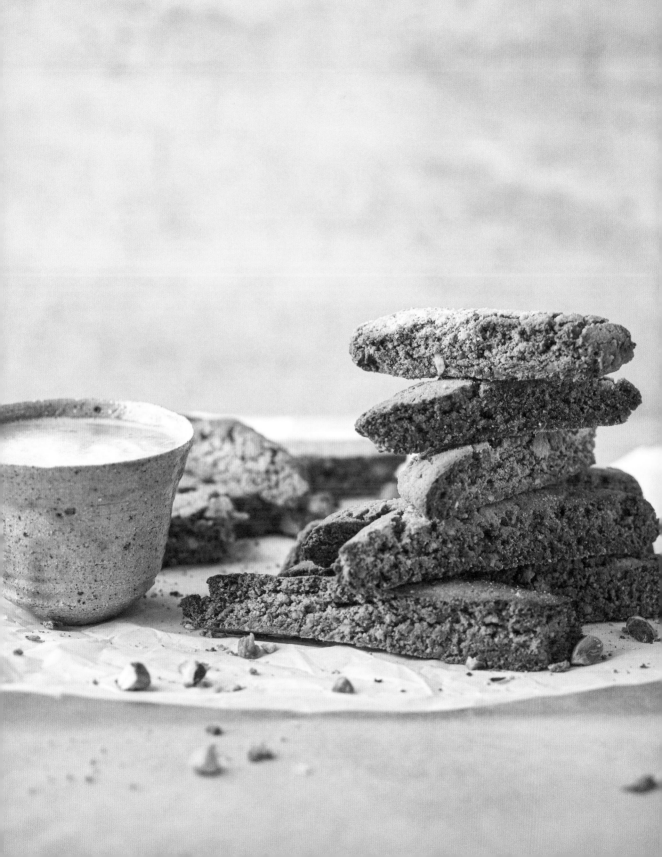

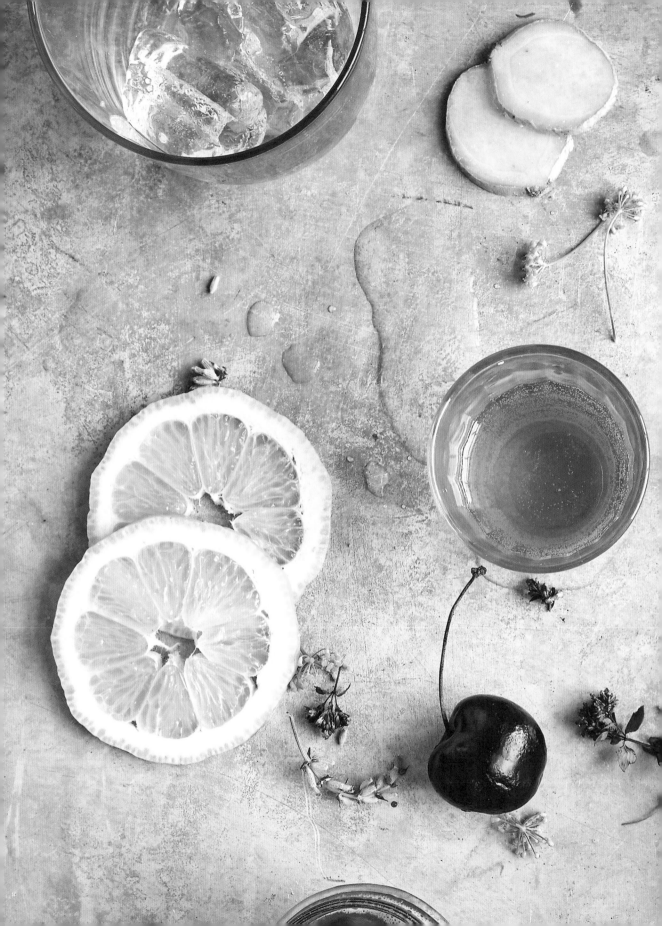

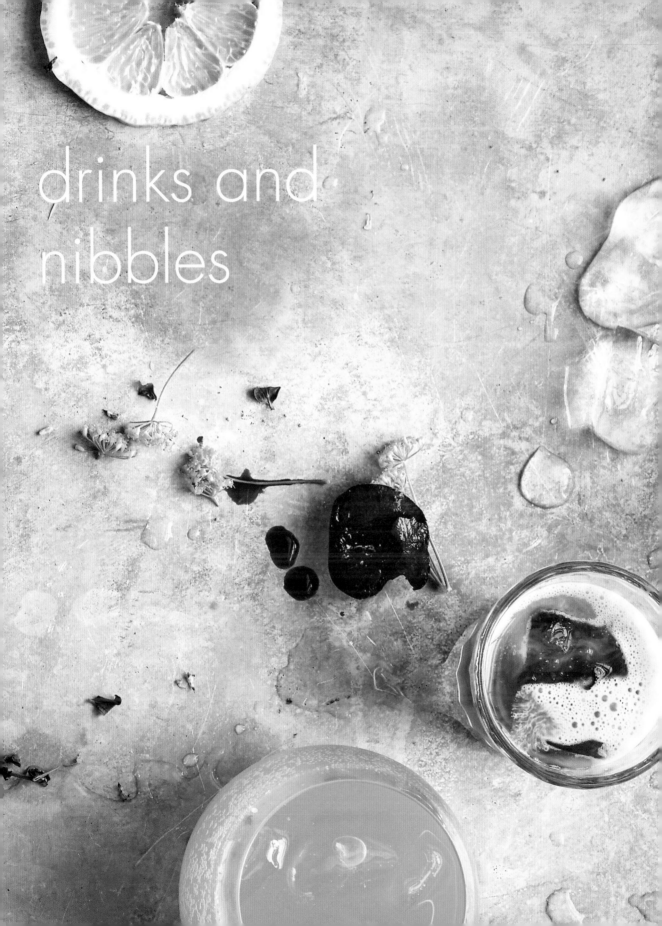

drinks and
nibbles

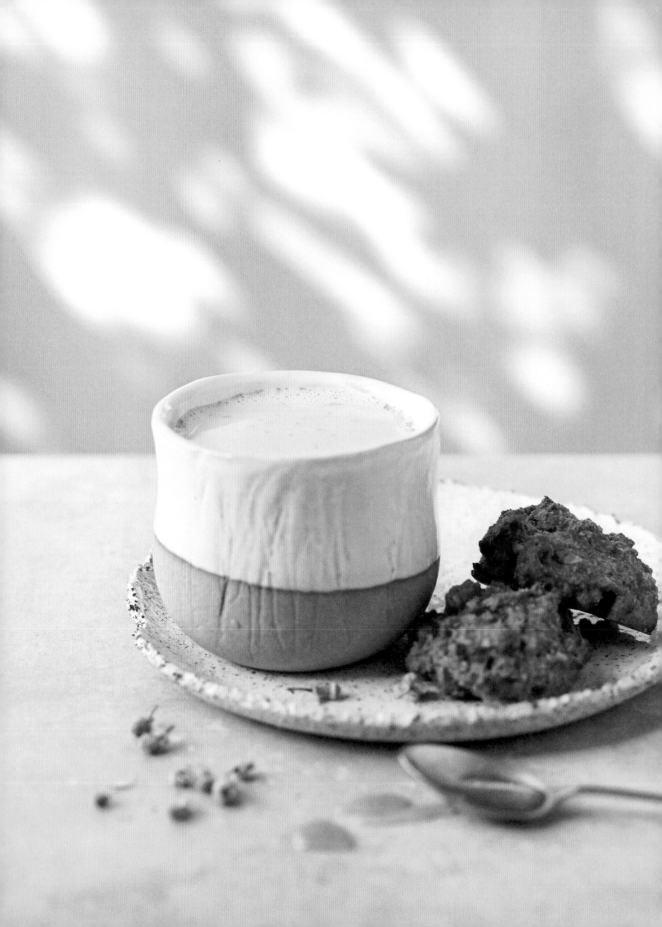

maca mocha

Maca mocha uses ground chicory as a coffee substitute. It's great for coffee lovers like myself who fancy something after dinner that won't keep them awake. Chicory is also high in inulin, a type of prebiotic that helps to feed the microbiome. Maca is made from the dried root of a South American plant that has been used for centuries for its stamina building and stress management properties, but in all honesty I think it just gives a rich and malty flavour to the drink.

serves 2

2 tablespoons maca powder
2 tablespoons ground chicory
2 teaspoons unsweetened cocoa powder
½ teaspoon vanilla extract
400ml milk of your choice – I think unsweetened oat milk works best

Put the maca, chicory, cocoa and vanilla into a small bowl and add enough of the milk to create a paste. Continue to gradually add milk, stirring until you have a thick liquid (by which time you will have used about two thirds of the milk). Pour this into a small saucepan and gently heat, stirring and gradually adding the remaining milk until it is warm, not boiling. Pour into mugs and enjoy!

sweet dreams milk

This idyllic nightcap – shown opposite with my yummy almond cookies (see page 183) – will have you drifting off into the land of nod. Chamomile is renowned for its calming and sleep-inducing properties. Oats and honey both encourage the production of melatonin, the main hormone needed for healthy sleep, so simply sit back, sip and await a blissful night's sleep.

serves 1

175ml unsweetened oat milk
1 teaspoon honey
Pinch grated nutmeg
1 tablespoon dried chamomile flowers or a tea bag made with chamomile flowers

Put all the ingredients in a small saucepan and gently heat, taking care not to boil. If using dried flowers, use a tea strainer to pour the milk into a cup; if using a tea bag then just remove and pour into your cup.

yuzu whisky highball

A life well spent wouldn't be complete without a few great cocktails along the way. Yuzu juice tastes like a combination of orange and grapefruit; it's a remarkable citrus flavour that goes perfectly with the whisky (I used Nikka Whisky from The Barrel). Here's to the longevity of your microbes!

serves 1

2 tablespoons yuzu juice
Generous squeeze lemon juice
55ml whisky
100ml sparkling mineral water
¼ teaspoon bicarbonate of soda

Add ice to a cocktail shaker then add the yuzu, lemon juice and whisky, and shake. Pour into a long glass over ice. Top up with the sparkling water, add the bicarbonate of soda and give a gentle stir.

mezcal booch mule

I believe a well-chosen tipple now and again is part of the joy of life. Enjoyed mindfully and responsibly it can also help to give frazzled nerves a bit of respite. In this recipe I've put a fermented spin on a classic by using ginger kombucha instead of ginger beer and mezcal rather than the usual voddy. You might have to shop around to source these but it's well worth it.

serves 1

50ml shot of mezcal (or tequila)
Juice of 1 lime
200ml ginger kombucha

Add the mezcal shot to a glass or cup with a couple of ice cubes. Squeeze in the lime juice and top with the kombucha.

honey sesame coconut chips

Preparing these delightful chips can bring a bit of gentle awareness back into your day. And of course coconut is bountiful with healthy fats that help to support both the gut and the brain.

makes approx. 4 servings

225g coconut chips
3 tablespoons black sesame seeds
3 tablespoons runny honey (or maple syrup for a vegan version)

Preheat the oven to 150°C/Gas 2. Line a baking tray with baking parchment.

Put the coconut chips and sesame seeds in a large bowl and stir to mix. Add the honey and stir to coat evenly. Transfer to the baking tray and bake for 20–25 minutes, checking after 20 minutes. Leave to cool for 25–30 minutes.

Store in an airtight container in the fridge to keep them crisp for up to 3–4 days.

panch phoran parsnip crisps

Parsnips are an excellent source of fibre, to support the microbiome, and these spicy, sweet crisps are perfect with an aperitif.

makes approx. 4 servings

1 tablespoon organic butter or ghee
2 parsnips, peeled and sliced into 2–3mm discs
1 tablespoon panch phoran spice blend
A few generous pinches sea salt.

Preheat the oven to 150°C/Gas 2. Line a baking tray with baking parchment.

Melt the butter or ghee in a large frying pan, add the parsnips and spice blend and stir-fry for 3–4 minutes until golden.

Spread the slices on the baking tray, sprinkle with the salt and bake for 1 hour. Store in an airtight container.

Al's white Russian

With all of the challenges that our brain and microbiome have to face, sometimes it is nice to kick back with a delicious cocktail. White Russian being one of my brother's favourites, I decided to put a bit of a spin on this and use cold brew coffee; if it's not available you can use regular coffee and just let it cool. The White Russian is served here with my Honey Sesame Coconut Chips (recipe on page 195).

serves 1

40ml vodka

2 tablespoons cold brew coffee

150ml unsweetened cashew milk or Jersey or Guernsey full fat milk

1 teaspoon maple syrup

¼ teaspoon vanilla extract

Add ice to a cocktail shaker then add the vodka and coffee and shake. Pour into a tumbler.

Put the milk, maple syrup and vanilla into a measuring cup and whisk. Slowly add the milk to the coffee and vodka mix. Sit back and sip!

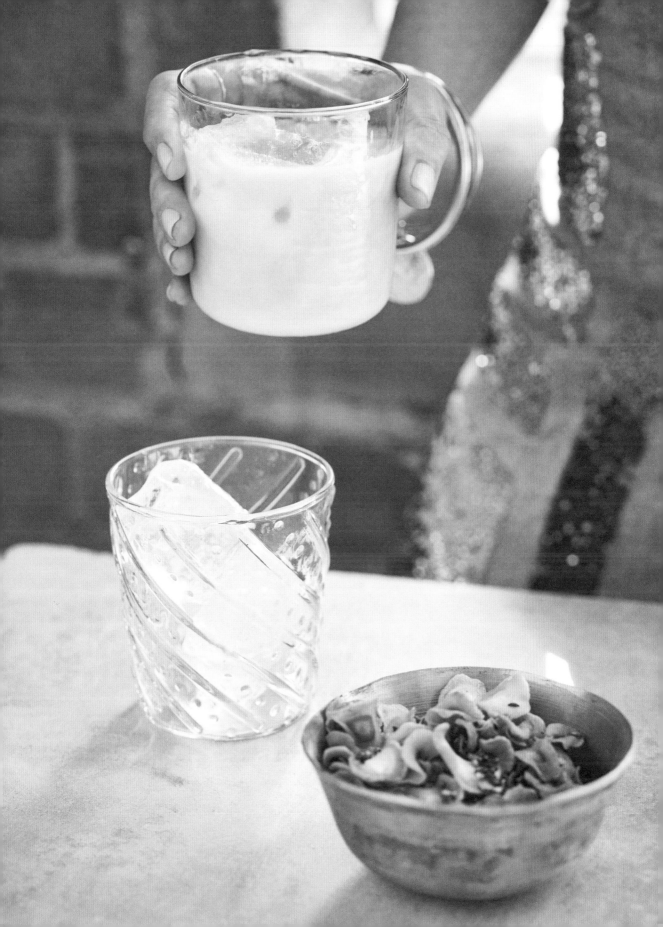

a few ferments

I'VE MENTIONED FERMENTED foods, and their associated benefits for our gut health, many times throughout the book. While you can buy ready-made fermented foods (check they are unpasteurised, though), there is something truly fascinating about witnessing the process of microbes transforming food into ferments. And of course it's so satisfying, too. The recipes in this section can help guide you on your journey of fermentation, whether you're a complete novice or want to expand your repertoire. The process may seem a little dauting initially, and the idea of microbes multiplying might require a little time to get your head around, but I promise that once you start you'll be hooked. Rest assured, the recipes don't require a lot of hands-on time – it's much more to do with patience, as you allow microbes to get to work. And it is worth the wait...

I've also included a basic homemade bone broth recipe at the end of this section as it's a valuable basic recipe for lots of purposes.

sauerkraut

Sauerkraut is the result of salt acting on cabbage to release juices that feed beneficial lactic acid bacteria so that they can flourish. Being of Polish descent, I was born and raised with lots of it! This is one of the easiest ferments to make so it's a great one to start with. Usually it requires just two ingredients – cabbage and water – but this is my grandfather's recipe and he liked to spice things up with some chilli and caraway. If you're not new to ferments feel free to riff on this as you like with your preferred flavours.

Note: it is important to use filtered water when you make vegetable ferments as tap water can contain compounds that can inhibit microbial growth.

makes about 400g (one large jar)

kit

Large glass or ceramic bowl
Large wide jar with lid
Paper weight or small jar
Some muslin cloth
Rubber band

ingredients

1 medium cabbage (you can use white or red or a mix of the two)
2 tablespoons mineral-rich salt
1 tablespoon caraway seeds
½ red chilli, deseeded and finely chopped (optional)

method

Clean everything to give the beneficial bacteria the best chance to thrive. Clean your hands thoroughly, too.

Shred the cabbage into very thin strips and place in a large bowl. Add the salt and massage thoroughly (to help release liquid from the cabbage) until you get a pool of liquid in the bottom of the bowl. This usually takes around 15–20 minutes or so. Now add the caraway seeds and chilli, if using.

Place the cabbage in the jar and pack down as much as possible. Top with the liquid from the bowl so that it completely covers the cabbage (if there is not enough, then mix some filtered water with a little salt and add that). Use a paper weight or small jar to keep the cabbage submerged.

Cover the jar with muslin cloth, secured with a rubber band, so the kraut can breathe. Press down every few hours, making sure the liquid covers the cabbage.

After 24 hours, cover the jar with a lid and keep it at room temperature for a further 5 days minimum. Remember to 'burp' your jar every day to release gas by just lifting the lid. Your kraut should then be ready to eat, but you can leave it longer for extra flavour and fermentation. When it tastes the way you want it to, store it in the fridge.

sourdough starter

This is what you need to begin making sourdough, which we will come on to next. It might seem a long process to get from start to finish but good things come to those who wait. For the flour, I've suggested organic since it has more of the naturally present bacteria and yeasts so it tends to ferment quicker, and, in my opinion, it gives a nicer flavour, but you can use regular flour if you prefer.

kit

Jar with a lid – make sure you clean this thoroughly before you begin
Small wooden spoon or plastic spatula

ingredients

50/50 mix of organic wholemeal bread flour and white bread flour (not self-raising)
Filtered warm water

method

First things first, try to keep your timings consistent as this is one of the key things needed to create a healthy starter. Get into a routine so you remember to feed your starter. Set a timer on your phone if you need or just do it as soon as you wake up and then right before bed from day four onwards. Here's the feeding schedule:

Day One – First thing in the morning put 50g of the flour in the jar and add 50ml of lukewarm water (around 26°C – use a thermometer if you need to). Mix well with your wooden spoon or spatula. Place the lid on loosely as the starter needs to breathe. Place in a dark and relatively warm place (somewhere around 20–25°C which is normal room temperature) for 24 hours.

Day Two – At the same time in the morning as day one, discard all but 1 tablespoon of the mixture and feed as before with 50g flour mix and 50ml lukewarm water. Pop it back in its cosy spot.

Day Three – As per day two.

Day Four At the same time in the morning, discard some mixture as per day two to leave 1 tablespoon then feed with the same 50g flour mix and 50ml water. Repeat this 12 hours later in the evening so you are giving the starter two feedings per day.

Day Five to Day Seven – Repeat Day Four exactly.

As you move through the days you should see the starter double in size. Don't expect there to be tons of activity in the first day or so, but as the days progress you will see some bubbles appearing. You may also notice a rather strong yeasty, sour smell. This is part of the process so don't freak out. It should settle down soon enough so perseverance is part of this. If you get something called a 'hooch', which is a layer of water, simply drain it off.

On day eight you should have a starter ready for baking. As few people bake every day, store your starter in the fridge. Allow at least one hour after your last feed before doing so and try to feed it on a weekly basis while it is in the fridge, using the same method above. You probably won't need to discard each week, as the temperature in the fridge will slow the fermentation down a lot. When you do decide to bake you'll need to give the starter a couple of feeds beforehand so consider taking it out of the fridge the day before you decide to bake a loaf and feed twice that day.

sourdough

Sourdough does take time to make but the end result tastes exceptional, gives a real sense of achievement and helps to nourish our gut microbiota. The distinctly sour flavour is largely due to the work of lactic acid bacteria in the fermentation process. During this process microbes essentially 'pre-digest' proteins such as gluten, as well as enhancing the bioavailability of nutrients in the bread itself. This is why sourdough can often be better tolerated by those who might ordinarily struggle with commercially made loaves. Furthermore, sourdough provides fibre for our gut microbiota and as such acts as a prebiotic to enhance numbers of our own resident beneficial bacteria. It's a 'win–win' for our taste buds and for the generous 'meal' it gives our gut microbes.

kit

Large mixing bowl

Banneton proving basket

Cast iron casserole dish with lid

Sharp bread knife to slash the dough

Scraper

ingredients

100g sourdough levain (made with starter – see page 200)

100g organic wholemeal flour

400g organic white flour

10g sea salt

50g rice flour

method

If your starter is in the fridge, take it out the day before and feed it in the morning and evening. (If you have just made it then it is good to go already.) The following morning, start making your levain. Take 1 tablespoon of the starter and put it in a jar. Mix with 50g 50/50 flour mix and 50ml lukewarm water – just as you would feed your starter. Leave in a warm spot for around 4 hours.

An hour before your levain is due to finish, mix all the flour with 325ml of water in a large bowl. Leave this flour mix in a warm spot next to the levain.

After you have left the levain for around 4 hours, it's time to give it a float test: take a tablespoon of the levain and drop it into some water – it should float. If it doesn't then you need to leave it a bit longer and test again.

Once ready, add 100g of the levain to the flour mix. Dimple this with your fingers into the dough to evenly distribute it. Leave for 15 mins. Now sprinkle over the salt and pour over 25ml of water. Mix well into the dough using the same dimpling technique. Lift and fold your dough over on itself four times at the different compass points, so north, east, south and west.

Repeat this lifting and folding, also giving it a gentle stretch, every 30 minutes for four sets. Be gentle as you don't want to tear the dough but you do want to create strength.

Shaping requires a confident attitude so don't spend too much time thinking about it. Lightly flour the surface you are working on and your hands and, taking the dough from underneath, move it onto the work surface and shape it into a ball. Cup the dough and drag it towards you. Turn and repeat two or three more times but don't overdo it. The dough should be firm and round.

Flour the inside of the banneton or, if you don't have one, use a large mixing bowl and a floured tea towel. Carefully lift the shaped dough into the banneton. Put in the fridge to prove overnight.

In the morning, preheat the oven to 230°C/Gas 8 and place a cast iron casserole dish with a lid inside the oven for at least 30 minutes before you start the actual bake. Take the dough out of the

fridge and turn onto enough parchment paper to just cover the bottom of the dough. Score along the top of the dough with a bread knife.

Remove the now VERY hot casserole from the oven and take off the lid. Place the dough (on the parchment) carefully into the casserole and replace the lid. Bake for 30 minutes. Remove the lid, reduce the temperature to 200°C/Gas 6 and bake for a further 20 minutes.

Remove from the oven and the casserole and allow to cool fully before slicing and enjoying! It will last a few days, but if you think you won't eat it all by then you can always slice and freeze it.

kefir

Kefir is a fizzy fermented drink that, through the process of fermentation, creates a bountiful amount of myriad beneficial microbes for our gut. It can either be milk (dairy) or water-based, which we can then drink to our (and our gut's) delight! Genuine kefir, whether it is dairy- or water-based (I've included a recipe for both on the following pages), can only be made from live grains, not from packets or powder. Remember, as discussed in Chapter 6, fermented foods rely on live sets of microbes. Your grains will multiply as you continue to ferment, because you are feeding them, so you can share the 'culture love' and pass on grains to friends and family. If you decide to have a break or don't want to make kefir batch after batch, or if you go on holiday, you can chill your grains. The method for doing this is described in each of the recipes.

dairy kefir

Best described as a slightly fizzy version of yogurt, kefir contains a more diverse and richer collection of microbes. It also has distinctive tart taste to it, which can take a bit of time to fully appreciate, but once you do you'll find it rather delicious. Don't be put off by the weird-looking grains that you need to ferment the milk as this is the crucial part of creating something special. I prefer to use raw (unpasteurised and unhomogenised) dairy milk as this gives increased amounts and diversity of microbes, but don't worry if you can't get this as you will still be able to make an excellent kefir with full-fat organic milk. The best time to drink kefir is on an empty stomach in the morning as it then has a better survival chance to get to the gut before digestion kicks in.
Plus, it gets you into a nice routine for starting the day ahead.

kit

2 large glass jars, one with a lid
Wooden spoon
Small plastic strainer or sieve
Muslin cloth

ingredients

2 tablespoons live milk kefir grains
500ml raw (unpasteurised) full-fat milk or organic unhomogenised full-fat milk

method

In a clean glass jar add the kefir grains and top with the milk. Cover with a muslin cloth and leave in a warm place to ferment for 24 hours.

After this time, use a plastic strainer like a small sieve and a wooden spoon to strain the milk into another clean glass jar, keeping the grains in the strainer. It is important not to use a metal spoon or strainer as this can affect the bacteria.

Chill the strained kefir in the fridge ready for when you want to drink it or you can drink it at room temperature if you prefer. It will keep for up to 2 days in the fridge.

Give the jar that you have used to ferment a good rinse, using filtered water, and put the strained grains back in. Top up again with the same quantity of milk to keep the kefir grains alive and to start the process again. Repeat the process every day.

tip

If you want a break from making dairy kefir, top the grains with milk and store in the fridge for up to 7 days. For longer periods, you can pat the grains dry and store in an airtight container in the fridge or freezer. Just bear in mind that when you start fermenting again, they will need a couple of rounds to warm up.

water kefir

Water kefir is like 'champagne for the gut' since it contains myriad strains of beneficial microbes that have a real celebration when they arrive to 'party' with our own gut microbes. Like dairy kefir, it should be fizzy – and it works on similar-looking grains that are more translucent than dairy ones – but that's really where the similarities end. Rather than feeding on lactose, as in the case of dairy kefir, water kefir grains like to 'eat' straight-up sugar. Most of this sugar is gobbled up by the microbes so that it doesn't end up in the final drink itself. I think water kefir is great as a morning tonic or in the afternoon as a bubbly pick-me-up!

kit

2 large glass jars, with a lid
Glass or ceramic jug
Wooden spoon
Small plastic strainer or sieve
Muslin cloth

ingredients

600ml lukewarm filtered water
3 tablespoons cane sugar
2 tablespoons live water kefir grains
2 slices of fresh lemon
1 prune
30g fresh fruit and herbs of your choice, roughly chopped – I love strawberries with some basil in mine but you can have fun experimenting

method

Fill one of the jars with the water and add the sugar. Stir to dissolve. Allow to cool and add the kefir grains, lemon slices and prune. Cover with some muslin cloth and leave at room temperature for 24 hours. Give the water a taste at this point to make sure that it is tangy rather than sweet. If it is still sweet then you may need to leave it a bit longer (check after another 4 hours).

Once ready, strain the kefir water through a sieve into a jug. The grains and the prune will be in the sieve. You can put the grains into another large jar to start the process again if you are making another batch or you can store in the fridge (see later notes on storage). Discard the prune.

In your second large jar, add the fresh fruit (and herbs if using) and top with the strained kefir water from the jug. Cover tightly with the lid and leave at room temperature for 24 hours ('burping' the jar to allow the carbon dioxide gas out every 4–8 hours).

The fruit should have floated to the surface after 24 hours, at which point 'burp it' again before storing in the fridge. You can strain to remove the fruit before you put it in the fridge or leave it in if you want more infusion of the flavour.

tip

If you want a break from making water kefir, top the grains with water and a teaspoon of sugar and store in the fridge for up to 14 days. For longer periods, you can pat the grains dry and store in an airtight container. Bear in mind, though, that when you start fermenting again, they will need a couple of rounds to warm up.

organic bone broth

Making bone broth is slow process but it's worth it, as it provides lots of flavour that can be used as a base for soups, stews or simply enjoyed on its own. During simmering, compounds such as collagen, glycine and glutamine are released from the bones and ligaments. These compounds are important for maintaining healthy connective tissue in the body, including the health of the gut barrier, which helps to manage general inflammation. In bone broth they can be more easily absorbed by the body.

Ask your local butcher or source chicken carcasses at farmers' markets – just make sure that you use bones from organic poultry. You can also use other bones left over from a roast, or source these from your butcher, and simply follow the same method used for chicken bones.

makes 3–4 litres

ingredients

3kg organic chicken carcasses, or 1 whole chicken carcass left over from a roast

approx. 4 litres filtered water

3 tablespoons apple cider vinegar

1 large carrot

1 large red or yellow onion

1 garlic clove

1 large celery stalk

2 bay leaves

3 sprigs of fresh thyme

1 tablespoon black peppercorns

method

Place the chicken pieces in a large saucepan, add the water and vinegar and leave to stand for 20–30 minutes. The vinegar helps the nutrients in the bones become more readily available.

Thoroughly wash the carrot but don't peel it as there is a lot of nutrition in the skin; don't peel the onion or garlic, either. Roughly chop all of the vegetables and add to the pan along with the bay, thyme and peppercorns, making sure that the water covers the ingredients by a good 5cm.

Bring to a gentle boil then reduce the heat and simmer with a lid loosely covering the pan. Skim off and discard any foam that forms, and check roughly every 20 minutes in the first couple of hours, skimming as necessary. When skimming you can also make sure the ingredients are fully covered with water and top up if needed. Simmer gently for 6 hours.

Remove the chicken pieces (you can save any meat from the bones to add to a salad or sandwich). Pour the liquid through a fine strainer into a large glass bowl; you can put the bowl into a sink of cold water or ice to speed up the cooling process. It is important to ensure that the broth is fully cooled before transferring into storage jars, otherwise you will have a breeding ground for less friendly microbes. Cover the jars and store in the fridge for up to 5 days or in the freezer for up to 1 month.

14-day happy planner

THIS PLAN CAN help you to put my recipes, mindfulness suggestions and practical tips into action. See what works for you and tweak it as you prefer. If you can aim to repeat this, which means doing it for roughly a month, it will provide consistency and can help form and reset habits that you can adopt long term. Even if that's making up a weekly batch of granola, it is doing something positive for yourself, which is great. Having a happy thought or action to adopt each day is definitely a great thing to support a happy mind.

day	take 5 on rising	breakfast	lunch
1	Start your day with 5 minutes of deep breathing before you do anything like check your phone or emails	Salted Caramel Apples with yogurt	Kim-cheese Toastie
2	Set your alarm 5 minutes earlier and take extra time to sit and be present over this morning's breakfast. Waffles deserve dedicated time and attention after all	Waffle time! Try my trrri-fic Tiger Nut Waffles	Lentil, Tomato & Walnut Poached Egg Salad
3	Start the day by stretching out your body and give your mind space to breathe	Chestnut Porridge, Star Anise Pears & Chestnut Cocoa Cream	Sourdough, Ricotta, Figs & Nigella
4	Spend the first moments of the day writing down three things you are looking forward to today	Pecan Pie Granola with yogurt or milk	Sourdough, Ricotta, Figs & Nigella
5	Think about a friend or family member that you haven't seen for a while and start the day by sending them a nice message	Cumin Scramble & Courgette Waffles	Smoked Mackerel with Caponata
6	Get some dedicated daylight exposure today, ideally first thing in the morning to support a better sleep–wake cycle	Seasonal Fruit Fool	Greens & Grains with a Miso Mustard Dressing

dinner	practical tip	happy act or thought	closing the day
Za'atar Spiced Lamb Burger	Make double the quantity of burgers to have tomorrow night too	Do something fun today	Have a relaxing bath before you begin your meditation tonight
Za'atar Spiced Lamb Burger	Pack your lunchbox with the ingredients you need to assemble tomorrow's easy and delicious lunch	Look up rather than down. You never know what opportunities and people you may attract	Burn a candle to bring warmth and light into your evening
Roasted Smoky Squash, Greens & Goats' Cheese Bowl	Find time today to make the Pecan Granola and fill your kitchen with the beautiful aromas of it baking	Give generously to others, whether it's time, attention or money. Kindness breeds kindness	Apply massage hand cream deeply into the centre of your palms to relieve stress from the day
Baked Bream, Fennel & Tomatoes	Make your caponata tonight ready for tomorrow's lunch and freeze the rest for next week	Be ready to receive the unexpected positives in your day	Listen to some classical or other soothing music this evening
Ras El Hanout Aubergine & Carrots	Boil half a dozen eggs to keep in the fridge for the week ahead for lunches or snacks	Go out for a walk today, leaving your phone at home	Spend time with a good book before you go to bed
Harissa Chicken with Lemon & Pomegranate	Get your baking hat on and bake the buckwheat bread for two lunches – take what you need, slicing and freezing the rest	Appreciate the little things like a hot bath or a warming cup of tea	Switch your phone off an extra hour before you go to sleep

day	take 5 on rising	breakfast	lunch
7	Spend a bit more time thoughtfully making your bed this morning – remember your bed is your sanctuary so show it gratitude for the comfort it gives you	Pecan Pie Granola with yogurt or milk	2 slices Buckwheat, Caraway & Pumpkin Seed Bread with 2 organic boiled eggs and baby spinach leaves
8	Have warm water with lemon juice upon rising and take some time to gently sip and reflect before you begin your day	Peanut Butter & Cinnamon Overnight Oats	2 slices Buckwheat, Caraway & Pumpkin Seed Bread with smoked salmon or hummus and rocket leaves
9	Set an intention to guide your thoughts and actions for the day ahead: for example, being more understanding of others or having a more light-hearted attitude to whatever life throws at you today	Seasonal Fruit Fool	Asparagus, Feta, & Pea Frittata
10	Music sings to the soul – put on a favourite track and start your day on a positive high literally shaking off any stress	Fig, Honey & Almond Oat Bakes	Asparagus, Feta, Pea & Frittata
11	Start your day with 5 minutes of meditation as well as your daily closing practice	Fig, Honey & Almond Oat Bakes	Hap-pea Soup

dinner	practical tip	happy act or thought	closing the day
Wild Salmon, Pak Choi & Leeks with Sesame Ponzu Sauce	Remember to soak your oats tonight ready for tomorrow's brekkie	You can do it!	Have some Sweet Dreams Milk to help support deeper ZZZs
Tempeh Tacos	Make your frittata this evening so that you can have it for lunch tomorrow and double the amount you need so that you can get two lunches for the price of one!	Be extra kind to yourself today	Write down three positive things that have happened today
Monkfish Nuggets with Sweet Potato Fries	Make a batch of Fig, Honey & Almond Oat Bakes for a couple of easy breakfast options and/or if you need a little snack – freeze what you don't need	Open your heart to receiving and giving love	Put out the clothes that you are going to wear tomorrow – to free up the headspace to ease yourself into your day
Pistachio-crusted Lamb Cutlets, Artichokes & Mint	I reckon tonight's dinner scene deserves a cocktail – pick one from the book or enjoy a nice glass of wine	Be happy with who you are and forget what you think you should be	Give your gut some hands-on love and attention with an abdominal massage, working in an anti-clockwise direction for 5–10 minutes
Crispy Prawns with Chilli Fennel & Smoky Paprika Dip	Don't forget to make your Bakewell Bircher before you hit the pillow tonight	Take things at your own pace	Spritz your pillow with lavender mist to support a deeper sleep

day	take 5 on rising	breakfast	lunch
12	Begin to create a book of inspirational quotes that resonate with you and that you can pick up and read to set the tone for the day ahead – start today with one quote that you feel resonates with your values	Bakewell Bircher	Kim-cheese Toastie
13	Walk to work, get off the bus or tube one stop earlier ... whatever it takes to get an extra 5 minutes walking time to help shake off any worries before you begin your day	Peanut & Miso Muffins	Portobello Egg 'Muffin'
14	Tap into the energy of the morning sunrise and use it to inspire your first thought for the day ... and make it a good one!	Peanut & Miso Muffins	Beet Kebab Couscous Bowl with Beet Borani

dinner	practical tip	happy act or thought	closing the day
Miso & Honey-Glazed Chicken Thighs	Let's make some muffins! Bake a batch of the Peanut & Miso Muffins that you can have for a couple of breakfasts – freeze any you don't need	Believe in yourself	Write down three things that you are grateful for today
Beet Kebab Couscous Bowl with Beet Borani	Make double the quantity of the beet kebabs and borani tonight to have for lunch tomorrow	Let go of the people and stuff that don't make you feel good	Spend an extra 5 minutes this evening on your preferred mindful practice which could be breathing exercises or meditation
Jungle Curry	Plan your shopping order for the next week	Happiness comes from within	Take time to reflect over what may have shifted positively for you over the past 14 days and perhaps the habits and thoughts that can remain a constant for you

ingredients guide

THIS SECTION IS DESIGNED to give you a bit more knowledge around some of the specific foods and food groups that are included in many of the recipes and throughout the book itself. My overall premise is that we should embrace *all* foods as part of an inclusive and positive approach to eating well, and the aim of this guide is to help you do that. Obviously this excludes those with allergies to certain foods, such as coeliacs, but not self-diagnosed food intolerances. This can often result in major food groups being unnecessarily excluded when the issue may be the quantity and/or specific type of food, or simply a gut that is generally struggling. It is always best to work with a qualified nutritionist if you suspect that certain foods are contributing to your gut symptoms.

dairy

Dairy has a lot of nutritional benefits, including providing calcium for bone health; and in the case of fermented foods, such as yogurt, kefir and cheese, it can provide a source of bacteria believed to be beneficial for our gut health. That said, some people do experience digestive symptoms as a result of eating dairy, which could possibly be due to lactose intolerance and/ or reaction to specific casein proteins.

If you experience a reaction to regular milk, you might find that ingesting fermented dairy – in the form of yogurt, dairy kefir (see page 203 for the recipe) or traditional cheese – doesn't cause the same reaction. This is because the fermentation process involved in producing these forms of dairy mean that much of the lactose and the proteins are broken down and essentially 'eaten' by microbes. With milk, which is not fermented, swapping to Guernsey/Jersey milk, which is predominant in what are called A2

beta-casein proteins, as opposed to the A1 beta-casein proteins that are dominant in most other cow's milk, might help. It has been suggested that this is due to the fact that human breast milk contains only A2 beta-casein proteins and therefore A2 cow's milk is more suited to our own profile. Goat and sheep dairy products are also predominant in A2 beta-casein proteins.

More generally, sourcing milk that is unhomogenised, which means it doesn't undergo high-pressure processing, can also help, as the structure of the milk is not manipulated, potentially making it easier to tolerate for those who experience digestive issues. I also think that buying organic dairy, or buying directly from farmers that you know practise fair principles, is essential as it is in some part contributing to a more ethical and sustainable farming system. I use Guernsey whole organic milk from **The Estate Dairy**, **Hurdlebrook** or **Abel & Cole** in my recipes and at home, but you can easily source this type of milk in your supermarket, online or locally.

When it comes to yogurt, many people find it easier on their gut than milk, because of the fermentation process mentioned above. Nevertheless, if you do find that cow's milk yogurt gives you some tummy troubles then perhaps try sheep or goat yogurt instead. Ricotta, which is a soft cheese, can also be tolerated by those who react to the casein proteins in cow's milk since it is made from whey.

On the cheese front, as a general guide, if you are heating it up or cooking with it, there is no real need to look for those made from raw or unpasteurised milk; however, if you are eating it in its raw state then you will get a wider variety of bacteria in cheeses made from unpasteurised milk.

Of course, there are those who choose not to have any dairy in their diet, due to allergies or for ethical reasons, which is fair enough. Plant-based milks can work as a substitute in some instances, although they don't have the same nutritional profile and unless fortified will lack crucial nutrients such as calcium. If this applies to you then ensure that you get rich, plant sources of calcium into your diet if you are not using a fortified plant-based milk. I use **Plenish** organic almond milk and **Oatly** whole oat milk in my recipes and as my recommended sources.

bread

Coeliac disease aside, which is a diagnosed allergy to gluten, there has been an unfortunate trend to exclude gluten and/or wheat from the diet without careful thought. Some of the digestive symptoms experienced after eating bread could in fact be attributed to the added ingredients that are present in many of our supermarket loaves, such as preservatives that can disrupt the microbiome. It could also be linked to the type of commercial yeast used, as that can also create digestive symptoms in certain individuals. Breads that are created using a natural fermentation process, as is the case with sourdough, can be easier to digest for many people who have issues with wheat or gluten. The slow process used to prepare sourdough is actually how we made bread for millennia. So I would encourage you to invest in good quality fresh sourdough that is made with just flour and salt or, even better, make it yourself (see page 201 for the recipe) – it can be more cost-effective and has the added benefit of filling your home with the glorious aroma of baking bread. It's also pretty simple once you get the knack and get into a regular routine of making it.

meat

Eat less and eat better is my personal philosophy when it comes to eating meat. Buying organic grass-fed or free-range meat not only equates to higher nutritional value, but it also contributes to better welfare standards for the animals. It might be more expensive but it is worth the extra pennies, and to counterbalance the added cost I also encourage you to have at least two to three meat-free days per week. Sourcing organic meat is relatively easy; you might also have local farmers who you can buy direct from – farmers' markets can be great for this and are generally more cost-effective. A responsible supplier that really takes care and attention over their farming is **Daylesford Organic** **www.daylesford.com** and you can purchase their meat online. Another good online stockist is **Coombe Farm Organic** **www.coombefarmorganic.co.uk**

I also use organic bone broth in a few recipes, as well as discussing its value to the gut on page 63. You can make this yourself (see page 205) or you buy it in your supermarket. My personal favourite is **Borough Broth** **www.boroughbroth.co.uk**

sweeteners

As with any other food, there is no need to entirely exclude sugar from the diet in order to be 'healthy'. At the end of the day, all types of sugar are pretty much the same. You might find more trace minerals in those such as maple syrup or coconut sugar but it equates to the same thing. When choosing a sweetener I tend to go for flavour over anything else, and what will best suit the recipe. Honey is one sweetener that has been used for millennia for its renowned healing properties, but this refers to raw or unpasteurised honey that hasn't been heat-treated so that it retains all of its nutritional benefits, including enzymes and antioxidants. Raw honey is often more opaque and less syrupy than some of the supermarket versions. If you are eating it without heating – i.e. you are not cooking with it – and you want to max on some of these added benefits then it's best to plump for the raw/unpasteurised stuff. I reckon it tastes much nicer too. And if you can source local honey and support nearby bee keepers, who are contributing massively to the welfare of the bees, even better.

wine

I love a glass of wine, and in the past few years have made a distinct effort to … erm 'study' it, all in the purpose of research of course! While we are all becoming more interested in the source of our food, we might not pay the same attention to the wine we drink. In fact, wine can harbour quite a lot of 'added ingredients' that you have probably never remotely considered. Moreover, grapes can be grown and harvested without any environmental and/or ecological concern. One solution? Natural wines. They don't have a specific label so they do require a bit of sourcing, but once you taste them it is hard to go back. Unlike some of the cheap, mass-produced wines – which rely on lower quality grapes that are sprayed with chemicals, and that have lots of added sugar – natural wines are made with grapes that are grown organically and with minimal intervention. The grapes are also picked when they are ready and not when it suits the 'production line' of the vineyard. Natural wines are also unfiltered and free of added

(as opposed to naturally occurring) sulphites. The caveat is that you may just get a bit of sediment with your sip. To read more about this and to source these wines go to **Pull the Cork www.pullthecork.co.uk** – founder James D. Nathan has also given some of his top wine pairings with some of my recipes.

quality ingredients and where to find them

flours

BUCKWHEAT You can find this pretty easily in most big supermarkets now, but if you need to you can also source it online. I like the **Rude Health** one, which also happens to be sprouted.

GRAM This is sometimes called Besan flour. It is milled from small chickpeas and is traditionally used in a lot of Indian dishes. You can source it in many supermarkets or online. I use **Dove Farm** gram flour in my recipes.

TIGER NUT I use this in some of my recipes as its brimming with prebiotic fibre that helps to feed microbes in the gut. It isn't that readily available but you can check out **The Tiger Nut Company** and order online **www. thetigernutcompany.co.uk**

CHESTNUT This is high in fibre and a great alternative for those who need to avoid gluten and/or want a grain-free flour. My go-to brand is **Amisa** chestnut flour, which you can find in health food stores or online.

COCONUT Also high in fibre and a little goes a long way. You can find this in some supermarkets and most health food stores. I like **Tiana** organic coconut flour.

sprouted grains

When grains have been sprouted it releases more of their nutritional potential and makes them easier on the gut so, if you have the option, go for these. Soaking also does a similar thing, and if you don't have sprouted grains to hand then soaking them is a good idea. This can break down and minimise substances in grains that are the plants' 'natural defence', and the ones that can create digestive discomfort for some people.

OATS **Rude Health** sprouted oats can be found in bigger supermarkets or look for **Sun & Seed** or **Planet Organic** online **www.planetorganic.com**

BUCKWHEAT Have a look at **Planet Organic** or **Sun & Seed**.

BROWN RICE **Planet Organic** have an own-brand version of this.

activated nuts and seeds

In my last book, *Be Good to Your Gut*, I gave guidelines on how to soak and activate nuts and seeds. This releases more of their nutrition potential and helps with their digestibility. Activating nuts and seeds can be particularly useful if you are following an exclusive plant-based diet, because it means that you can optimise sources of protein, zinc and iron, which can often be lacking. However, I'm mindful that not everyone has the inclination to do this, so don't let this be an added stress for you if you don't want to do it.

If you want to soak and activate, then great, here's how to do it. Soak your nuts or seeds overnight with enough water to cover them well and add a pinch of salt. In the morning, rinse well and spread over a baking tray and heat in the oven on the very lowest setting. Check after 10 hours – they should be crunchy, but if not, pop in for a further 1–2 hours. Alternatively, use a dehydrator. Store once cooled. If you want to buy nuts and seeds that are already activated they are available, but they can be rather pricey.

condiments

Most of these can be found easily enough in supermarkets or online. I've included some of my top picks below.

TAMARI AND SOYA SAUCE Tamari is gluten free, but you can use traditional (and properly fermented) soya sauce instead of tamari if you don't have any issues with wheat/gluten. Soy sauce is one of the most widely used fermented foods. Check out **Tsuru Bishio**, which is aged in the traditional 'kioke' wooden barrels with multitudes of microbes to get to the delicious end product. Source this at **www.vallebona.co.uk/tsuru-bishio-aged-soy-sauce-by-yasuo-yamamoto/** Otherwise, and for a soy-free version, use coconut aminos such as **Coconut Secret**.

VEGAN MAYO Aquafaba mayo is made from the water left from soaking chickpeas, which makes it sustainable as well as egg- and dairy-free. Have a look at **Rubies in the Ruble** for this, which is available in many major supermarkets. They also do an outstanding ketchup.

GARLIC-INFUSED OLIVE OIL This is a great alternative to garlic cloves for those who find that eating garlic can cause a grumbling gut. I really like the one from **Seggiano,** which you can get at their online shop or Planet organic online or many nationwide delis. Otherwise you can easily find garlic-infused olive oil in most supermarkets.

spices

some of the spices I use in my recipes are not as easy to find, so here are some handy stockists.

LIQUORICE POWDER My favourite is by **Lakrids by Bulow**, which you can order online www.lakridsbybulow.co.uk or try **Sous Chef** www.souschef.co.uk

GROUND STAR ANISE For this and much more head to **Steenbergs**, which stocks almost every spice and dried herb you could ever need! www.steenbergs.co.uk

SUMAC You can also find this at Steenbergs or online from various stockists.

SPICE BLENDS I have used blends such as Panch Poran, Ras El Hanout and Za'atar in some of my recipes, which you might be able to find in your supermarket. If not then Steenbergs also stock these or **Ottolenghi** online shop www.ottolenghi.co.uk/shop

extra bits

COCONUT BUTTER Aka manna, this is basically the puréed flesh of the coconut rather than the oil and is therefore naturally sweet. Look for **Nutiva**, **Biona** or **Tiana**.

MATCHA POWDER My favourite matcha is from **Lalani & Co**. Find them online www.lalaniandco.com

BAOBAB POWDER I use **Aduna** in my recipes. You can find it in many big supermarkets or in health food stores.

GROUND CHICORY You can find this in most health food stores. I like **Chikko** or **Prewett's**.

TEMPEH Try to buy organic. **Tofoo** brand is available in many supermarkets.

MACA POWDER My go-to brand for this is **Naturya**, which you can find in many supermarkets or in health food stores.

YUZU JUICE You'll find this in some bigger supermarkets or you can easily order online.

COCOA POWDER My favourite is by **Valrhona**, which you can find at various online stockists, including www.souschef.co.uk

general online stockists

Daylesford www.daylesford.com
Planet Organic www.planetorganic.com
Ocado www.ocado.com
Steenbergs www.steenbergs.co.uk
Sous Chef www.souschef.co.uk

equipment

I use a Vitamix blender and a Magimix food processor. My spice/coffee grinder is Cuisinart.

tableware

Creating a 'rest and digest' atmosphere around your meals is just as important as the food on the plate in front of you when you are aiming to support a mindful gut–brain connection. Here are some of my top picks for places to source ceramics, linens and glassware. Also have a rummage in your local charity shops as you can find some real gems!

Kana London www.kanalondon.com
The Cloth Shop www.theclothshop.net
Skandihus www.skandihus.co.uk

resources

registered nutritional therapy and functional medical practitioners

BANT (British Association for Applied Nutrition & Nutritional Therapy) – use this website to find a registered nutritional therapist in your area **www.bant.org.uk**

CNHC (Complementary & Natural Healthcare Council) – a national voluntary regulator for complementary healthcare practitioners where you can find registered therapists local to you **www.cnhcregister.org.uk**

IFM (Institute for Functional Medicine) – the institute that coined the phrase 'functional medicine', which uses private lab testing for personalised treatments. You can find a certified practitioner at their website **www.functionalmedicine.org**

emotional, mental and cognitive health support organisations

MIND **www.mind.org.uk**

Rethink Mental Illness **www.rethink.org**

Alzheimer's Society **www.alzheimers.org.uk**

Parkinson's UK **www.parkinsons.org.uk**

National Autistic Society **www.autism.org.uk**

environmental and organic organisations

Farmers' markets – check out FARMA (National Farmers' Retail & Markets Association) to find your local markets and farm shops **www.farma.org.uk**

MSC (Marine Stewardship Council) – check this out to see how the sustainability and traceability of your fish choice racks up **www.msc.org**

PAN UK (Pesticide Action Network) for info on pesticides and how you can support more environmentally conscious initiatives **www.pan-uk.org**

The Soil Association is the UK's leading charity for healthy, sustainable and ethical farming practice and land use. Soil Association Certification is the UK's largest organic certification body – always look for their stamp when buying organic **www.soilassociation.org**

further reading

Here are some of my favourite stand-out books on gut health, emotional and mental wellbeing, microbes and fermentation and the simple pleasures of eating.

The Psychobiotics Revolution, John F. Cryan. Scott C. Anderson and Ted Dinan (National Geographic, 2017)

The Inflamed Mind, Edward Bullmore (Short Books Ltd, 2019)

The Source, Tara Swart (HarperOne, 2019)

Why We Sleep: The New Science, Matthew Walker (Penguin, 2018)

The Perfect Meal, Charles Spence (Wiley-Blackwell 2014)

Salt, Fat, Acid, Heat, Samin Nosrat (Canongate Books, 2017)

The Flavour Thesaurus, Niki Segnit (Bloomsbury, 2010)

How To Eat, Thich Nhat Hanh (Parallax Press, 2014)

The Art of Fermentation, Sandor Katz (Chelsea Green Publishing Co, 2012)

The Noma Guide to Fermentation, Rene Redzepi and David Zilber (Artisan Publishers, 2018) glossary

This A–Z glossary will help you familiarise yourself with some of the terms used throughout the book.

A

Adrenaline A stress hormone, also known as epinephrine, produced predominantly in the adrenal glands in response to a signal from the brain. It sends messages around the body to prepare for fight or flight, for example by increasing the heart rate and blood flow to the muscles.

Amino acids Used in every cell of the body, these compounds form the building blocks of protein, which is necessary for growth, repair and regeneration, and are vital for the production of things like enzymes, hormones and neurotransmitters. They also play a crucial role in storage and transportation of nutrients and metabolic processes. In the body there are twenty amino acids (known as standard amino acids), of which nine are 'essential' for humans, meaning that they cannot be made by the body and need to come from our food.

Amylase An enzyme that is produced in saliva glands and in the pancreas in order to break down carbohydrates into simple sugars.

Antibody/Antigen An antigen is a protein expressed by a bacteria or virus (usually on their cell surface) that is recognised by the immune system as 'foreign'; the immune system responds by producing an antibody (aka immunoglobulin). Some antibodies create an extreme response, such as the anaphylactic reaction of immediate swelling of the tongue or throat; other antibodies are working constantly to counteract pathogens in the gut.

Antioxidants Molecules found in a variety of foods, particularly vegetables, fruit, nuts and seeds, and also produced in the body, that help to protect cells against damage by oxidation. *See also* phytochemicals.

B

Bile A yellow/green liquid that is produced by the liver to help digest and absorb fats (it is stored in the gall bladder).

BDNF (brain-derived neurotrophic factor) a protein that supports the health and growth of neurons and overall cognitive function.

Bolus The small ball of food chewed in the mouth that then makes its way to the stomach.

Butyrate A short-chain fatty acid produced by microbes in the gut. It is the major source of energy for intestinal epithelial cells that line the gut and as such supports the intestinal barrier. It also has anti-inflammatory effects both in the gut and more systemically in the body. Also found in food sources such as raw milk, unpasteurised cheese, ghee and organic or cultured butter.

C

Cholecystokinin (CCK) The hormone that is released in response to fat from chyme as it enters the small intestine. It stimulates the release of digestive enzymes from the pancreas and emptying of bile from the gall bladder.

Chyme The mush of food in the stomach that makes its way to the small intestine.

Colony forming units (CFUs) Used in reference to probiotics, this indicates the number of live and actively viable microorganisms found in each dosage of a probiotic formula.

Commensal bacteria Bacteria that we co-exist with and have a mutualistic and beneficial relationship to.

Cortisol A stress hormone produced mostly in the adrenal glands in response to a signal from the brain. It sends messages around the body to prepare for fight or flight in the stress response.

Cytokines These are small proteins produced by immune cells and the gut microbiota that mediate communication between cells, including responses to inflammation and immune reactions.

D

Dopamine A neurotransmitter associated with pleasure and the reward system: in the gut, it helps to coordinate the contraction of muscles in the colon. Fifty per cent of overall dopamine is synthesised in the gut.

Dietary fibre The part of plant-based carbohydrates that we cannot digest but it makes its way to the large intestine to provide food and fuel for our gut microbes.

Dysbiosis a term used to describe an imbalance in the microbiome where potentially pathogenic microbes become higher in the numbers and may have a negative impact on the overall balance of microbes in the gut that can result in digestive and other gut related symptoms.

E

Enteric nervous system (ENS) The main way in which your gut 'thinks', the ENS consists of a highly intricate network of nerves embedded in the tissue lining the gut.

Enzyme A type of protein needed for chemical reactions throughout the body. Digestive enzymes are specific types of enzymes used to break down nutrients from our food.

G

GABA (gamma-amino butyric acid) The body's most important inhibitory neurotransmitter.

GALT (gut-associated lymphoid tissue) Lymphoid tissue of the gastrointestinal mucosa lines and protects the gut, which makes up 70–80 per cent of the entire immune system. GALT has a crucial role in managing what can pass out of the gut into the body, differentiating between harmless food proteins and microbes and those that can cause us harm, such as pathogens and toxins.

Ghrelin The 'hunger hormone' that targets the pituitary gland in the brain to say it's time to eat.

Glucagon This hormone plays a part in blood sugar regulation. It works with the liver to stimulate the conversion from glycogen to glucose, which is released to raise blood sugar levels when they drop too low. It also works in a process called 'gluconeogenesis', which is the production of new glucose from non-carbohydrate precursors such as amino acids.

Glucose A simple sugar that serves as the primary fuel for metabolic processes and energy in the body.

H

Homeostasis A state of balance and equilibrium in the body. Various systems work to maintain a constant internal environment that ensures the body operates optimally, including regulation of body temperature and volume of water in the body.

Hormones Chemical messengers produced by glands and specialised cells throughout the body. They communicate between organs and tissues on a wide range of activities, including digestion, respiration, sleep and reproduction.

I

Insulin The hormone that is released when we eat and blood sugar levels rise. In response, insulin signals glucose, our primary fuel, to be shuttled into cells ready for use. Insulin also controls excess stores of glucose and either stores it as glycogen in the liver or deposits it in fat tissue. It also communicates to the hypothalamus in the brain to suppress appetite so we know when to stop eating.

Intestinal epithelium The layer of cells that lines the small and large intestine and separates the gut (and the substances we have ingested) from the rest of the body.

Intestinal villi and **microvilli** Finger-like projections that line the small intestine; they assist with absorbing nutrients into the bloodstream.

L

Leptin A hormone produced by adipose (fat) tissues, it tells the brain when we are full and suppresses appetite.

Lipase The digestive enzyme that is responsible for breaking down fats.

Lipopolysaccharides (LPS) Toxic substances found in the cell membranes of certain types of bacteria that can create inflammatory responses in the body.

M

Melatonin A hormone primarily released by the pineal gland to regulate the sleep–wake cycle. It is also produced in the gut.

Microbiome The trillions of microbes *and* their genetic material, which live in and on us. The gut microbiome is now being considered an organ in its own right due to its far-reaching influence in the body.

Microbiota The collective population of microbes that live in and on us. This is mostly made up of bacteria but also contains fungi and other microorganisms. Technically they outnumber our own human cells, and the gut microbiota is the biggest collection, housing some trillions of microbes.

Microorganism or **Microbe** a tiny organism that can only be viewed through a microscope and collectively forms the microbiota. This could include bacteria, fungi and viruses. Some of these could be deemed 'beneficial', some superfluous, and others potentially pathogenic, depending on the type and amount.

Mitochondria are responsible for generating ATP (adenosine triphosphate), which is the prime source of fuel for cells to function

N

Neurons Cells in the nervous system that communicate to other cells using synapse connections. They receive sensory input from the external world and are responsible for sending muscular motor commands, transmitting information to glands and relaying signals to other neurons.

Neurotransmitters are 'chemical messengers' that communicate between neurons (nerve cells) and other cells (in nerves, muscles and glands). Neurotransmitters manage our thought processes and moods, as well as involuntary processes such as circulation and digestion.

O

Omega 3 A type of oil known as an essential fatty acid: 'essential' means they cannot be produced by the body and we need to get from the diet. They are crucial for the health of every cell membrane in the body and for brain health.

P

Pathogens Microbes that can potentially increase in number and activity in a way that may create disturbances and imbalances in the gut microbiota. *See also* dysbiosis

Pepsin The enzyme in the stomach that helps to break down protein.

Peptide YY (PYY) An appetite-suppressing hormone that the small intestine releases in response to eating. It slows down the passage of food to increase nutrient absorption.

Peripheral Nervous System (PNS) This system has two divisions: the somatic nervous system, which governs voluntary movements, and the autonomic nervous system (ANS), which manages involuntary processes such as breathing.

Phytochemicals or **phytonutrients** beneficial compounds found in plant-based foods that provide energy for microbes in the gut. Some examples could be flavonoids found in apples, onions and dark chocolate; lignans in sesame seeds; or curcumin in turmeric, to name just a few.

Prebiotics A food, or supplement, that contains certain types of fibre that have a more 'potent' feeding effect on specific beneficial microbes in the gut.

Probiotics Beneficial bacteria, and some yeasts, that have a positive role in the body. These are found naturally occurring in the gut and in fermented foods. However, it is typically a term used to refer to bacteria in supplementary form.

S

Serotonin A neurotransmitter, often described as our 'happy neurotransmitter' because it influences our mood and contributes to feelings of wellbeing. More than 90 per cent of our overall serotonin production comes from the gut.

Short-chain fatty acids (SCFAs) These are positive substances produced by microbes in the gut when they ferment dietary fibre. SCFAs provide energy for the cells in the lining of the gut and, more broadly, help to support the immune system, amongst many other roles.

Y

Yeast Microorganisms classed as part of the fungus family. Naturally occurring, or 'wild', yeasts have been used for millennia to make bread and beer. Other species of yeasts, such as *Candida albicans*, may affect the health of the microbiota. *See also* dysbiosis index

firmicutes 34
fish 141–51
    baked bream, fennel and
        tomatoes 150, *151*
    monkfish nuggets with sweet
        potato fries *146*, 147
    oily fish 67
    rainbow trout miso soba bowl
        148
    smoked mackerel with caponata
        and lemon yogurt dressing 142
    spicy wild salmon with celeriac
        saag aloo 143
    wild salmon, pak choi and leeks
        with sesame ponzu sauce 144,
        145
    see also anchovy
flavonols 66
flaxseed 90
flours 217
    see also specific flours
folic acid 23, 64
food, building a positive
    relationship with 15–16
food additives 67–70
food allergies 40, 71, 215–16
food exclusion 215–16
food intolerances 40, 70–2, 215
food restriction/elimination 70–2
fools, seasonal fruit fools 174, *175*
FOS *see* fructooligosaccharides
free radicals 66
'freeze' response 29
fries, monkfish nuggets with sweet
    potato fries *146*, 147
frittata, asparagus, feta and pea
    frittata 137
fructooligosaccharides (FOS) 62
fructose 69
fruit
    rainbow 66–7
    seasonal fruit fools 174, *175*
fungi 21

G

galactooligosaccharides (GOS) 62
gallbladder 20
GALT *see* gut-associated lymphatic
    tissue
gamma-amino butyric acid
    (GABA) 15, 23, 31–2, 35, 42, 54,
56, 74
Gandhi, Mahatma 44
ganglia 28
garlic
    chilli and garlic greens 170, *171*
    garlic-infused olive-oil 218
gas 45–6, 69, 77, 78
gastric juices 20
gelatin 63
genetics 24
Gershon, Michael 28
ghrelin 33, 56
ginger, sesame and ginger chicken
    noodle soup *108*, 109
glucosinolates 66
glutamate 32, 42
glutamine 63, 205
gluten 40, 216
glycine 63, 205
goats' cheese
    ras el hanout aubergine and
        carrots, goats' cheese and
        sumac tahini dressing *120*, 121
    roasted smoky squash, greens
        and goats' cheese bowl 129
GOS *see* galactooligosaccharides
grains 65
    see also specific grains
gram flour 217
granola, pecan pie granola 98
grazing 47
green bean 116, 148
greens 49
    five-spice pork burgers in chilli
        and garlic greens with coconut
        onion rings 170, *171*
    greens and grains with a miso
        mustard dressing 116, *117*
gut
    'anxious gut' 42
    definition 19
    'depressed gut' 42
    and digestion 19–21
    independence from the brain 15
    protective function 19
    and soul food 80–2, 84–6
    stressed 43, 44–50
    workings of the 18–26
gut acidity levels 45–6
gut barrier 21–2, 53, 65
    breaches 32, 33, 35, 38, 43, 45
    and butyrate 41
and cortisol 45
    and emulsifiers 70
    and the immune system 30
    and medication 74
    renewal 52
    and SCFAs 22, 32
    and vitamin C 49
    see also 'leaky gut'
'gut feelings' 13, 15, 36, 86
gut microbiome/microbiota 13, 15,
    18–22, *21*
    and babies 25–6
    and 'bad' gut microbes 24, 39, 42
    and cravings 34–5
    daily rhythms of the 53–5
    development 25–6
    diversity 39, 60
    eating well for 48–9, 59–72
    and the environment 73–9
    functions 22–3
    and genes 21–2
    and the gut–brain connection
        27–36
    inheritance 24–5
    and the large intestine 20–1
    and lifestyle 73–9
    and the mind 37–43
    and mitochondria 39–41
    and mood 37–43
    and pregnancy 25
    and sleep 51–8
    and soul food 85–6
    and stress 43, 44–50
    symbiosis/mutualism of 21,
        22–4
gut microbiome/microbiota
    28–30, 38
    see also microbiota-gut-brain
        axis
gut motility 20, 22–3, 28, 54
gut tranquillity 43
gut–brain connection 15–16, 18,
    21, 26, 27–36, 39, 80
    and antibiotics 74
    development 25
    and diversity of the microbiome
        39
    and the environment 73
    and lifestyle 73
    and sleep 53
    and soul food 86
    and stress 44–6

acknowledgements

Firstly, to Sarah, her David and the two 'monkeys' – you held me up and made me happy on days that felt insurmountable. So much love for you all.

To Nat, you are truly one in a million. Thank you for always being there for me, no matter what. And for bringing into the world such a beaming ray of sunshine, my little goddaughter Zara – you are a bundle of joy and positivity.

My brilliant mate Katy, I am so grateful to you for giving me strength and solidarity in the most challenging of times. To the amazing Alan and Dale – your unwavering love and support means so much. James T, you always bring me laughter and lightness. Thank you for being such a wonderful soul. And to Nat, you are strong, fearless and a bit crazy and I love you for all those reasons ... so lucky to have you in my life. To Jim, you have the biggest heart and the best hugs. You remind me that after rain comes a rainbow. Thank you for lifting me up emotionally and physically at a time when I needed it most.

My absolute wing-girl Emma, there is genuinely no way this book could have happened without you. To Aaron, the most talented web designer ever and some! Thanks for being our tech wizard. Georgie and the team at Beam, thank you for your consistent support and encouragement. You're the best.

Thanks to Barry and all at Symprove for continuing to drive the excitement, conversation and awareness around gut health – keep the momentum and the flag flying high! To Stephen, thank you for being a great friend and always championing me and my work ... here's to plenty more exciting projects ahead. And to Andrea, you are simply incredible. I can't wait to see where the future takes us together. To Suzy, it is an honour to work with you and the team at Psychologies, thank you for always supporting me. And to Kirsty and all at *Guardian* Masterclasses – thanks for continuing to give me such a brilliant opportunity (and stage!).

Thanks to the team behind the scenes – to my publisher Zoe and editor Jillian, who helped me create a book that exceeded expectations. It took longer than anticipated, but it was worth all the extra work. To my agent Katie, it's been a joy to have you on board with this book. To the wonderfully talented Nassima, thank you so much for beautifully capturing my dishes, and for putting me in such a positive light. And to Maria – your oat milk lattes are now legendary! To the dynamic duo in the kitchen – Rosie and Kitty, thank you for making my recipes look so awesome. And for the tastiest sourdough ever. Big shout-out to the styling team – Jenelle Thompson, Amalie Russell for Bobby Brown Cosmetics, Karishma G, Linda & Ida at Couverture & The Garbstore, and the lovelies at matchesfashion.com. Also a massive thanks to James D. Nathan, founder of Pull the Cork, for your wonderful wine pairings.

To my clients, who continue to inspire and push me onwards and upwards, I'm immensely proud to be part of your journey.

And last but by no means least, to my mum and dad: in the most heart-breaking and extreme moments of adversity you still manage to see the beautiful parts of life and the good in others. Your love and devotion have inspired me to keep on reaching for the stars and to dig deep for the soul and passion to write this book. I couldn't have done this without you two. And finally...

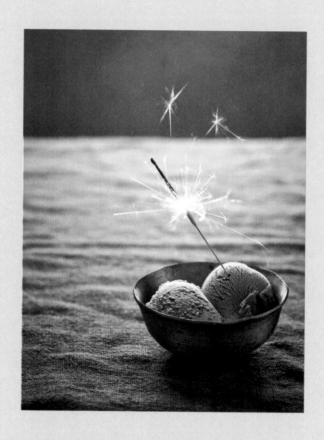

This book is dedicated to my
little brother Alex. I think of you
every day and hold you so close
to my heart. This is for you.
Love Sis x